Former corporate lawyer, co-founder of a successful software company and technology investor, David Gillespie is the best-selling author of the *Sweet Poison* books, *Big Fat Lies*, *Free Schools* and *Toxic Oil*. He lives in Brisbane with his wife and six children.

Also by David Gillespie

Free Schools

DAVID GILLESPIE

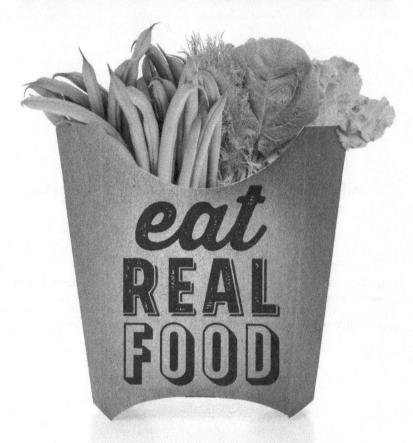

eat REAL FOOD

THE ONLY SOLUTION TO PERMANENT WEIGHT LOSS AND DISEASE PREVENTION

MACMILLAN
Pan Macmillan Australia

First published 2015 in Macmillan by Pan Macmillan Australia Pty Ltd
1 Market Street, Sydney, New South Wales, Australia, 2000

Cataloguing-in-Publication entry is available
from the National Library of Australia
http://catalogue.nla.gov.au

Typeset in Sabon by Kirby Jones
Printed by McPherson's Printing Group

The publishers and their respective employees or agents will not accept responsibility
for injuries or damage occasioned to any person as a result of participation in the
activities described in this book. It is recommended that individually tailored advice be
sought from your healthcare professional.

The author and the publisher have made every effort to contact copyright holders for
material used in this book. Any person or organisation that may have been overlooked
should contact the publisher.

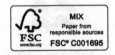

To Lizzie, Anthony, James, Gwen, Adam,
Elisabeth and Fin.

CONTENTS

CONTENTS

INTRODUCTION

In 2003 my wife, Lizzie, decided to make my life immeasurably harder. You see, she decided to make twins instead of our fifth child. We already had four kids under the age of eight, and adding twin babies to that was going to be about as much fun as being poked in the eye with several (six, probably) sticks. Weighing in at well north of 130 kilograms (I was afraid to see what the actual number was), I wasn't coping with the four we already had. It was time to reach for the panic button.

I hadn't amassed 40 extra kilograms (at least) on my waist overnight, I'd been working long and hard at it, accumulating a few extra kilograms every year of my adult life. Every now and then, I'd notice my (latest) favourite pants shrinking and decide to do something about it. This usually involved doing whatever fad diet I'd seen on the telly that week or joining a gym or walking the dog a lot. And these all worked. Every single time I applied willpower to the problem, my weight would drop and it would keep dropping for exactly as long as my willpower held out. In my case, that was usually about two weeks. Then I'd give up from the sheer effort of sustained self-control and the weight would come charging back (usually with a bit of interest). If willpower was the key to weight loss I was clearly doomed.

What I couldn't understand was why willpower was a necessary part of the equation. Every other species on the planet appeared to control its weight exactly the same way it controlled its height, on autopilot. Even when there was an abundance of food, other animals seemed to stop eating well before the point they gained 50 per cent of their body weight. The only exceptions to this rule appeared to be humans and any animal unfortunate enough to be fed by humans.

And even with humans, obesity appeared to be a problem that had only really become a bother in the last 200 years or so. As a species, we had successfully lived on this planet for at least a quarter of a million years, but only in the last 0.08 per cent of that time had we suddenly become lard-bottoms. If that time were represented as a day, we'd successfully avoided obesity for 23 hours and 57 minutes only to succumb at three minutes to midnight.

I didn't accept that we'd all suddenly developed some kind of mass loss of willpower. I didn't buy it because it didn't seem to be about timing. It seemed to be about exposure to the modern Western way of life. Or, as a biochemist friend once (half-jokingly) said, the strongest correlation with obesity and disease is speaking English. As soon as a people, be they Polynesian islanders or Chinese peasants, switched from their traditional way of life to a Western one, all the badness happened – everything from obesity to heart disease and every other chronic disease between. And this was a process that seemed to be happening all over the world to this very day. To buy the willpower story, I'd have to assume that something about traditional life gave us wills of steel and something about Western life was willpower-sapping. That would of course be nonsense. We are the same people with the same biochemistry and the same brains. Whether we can use a toaster instead of a fire or buy food rather than hunt it could not possibly alter our psychological make-up.

I figured that if I could get to the bottom of what it was about Western society that made us so fat – I was pretty sure it wasn't speaking English – I might find a way to avoid being so fat myself. So I hit the books. It quickly became apparent that exercise was not part of the answer. There were just too many studies showing that people have always been as lazy as their environment allows them to be. Traditional people exercised exactly as much as was required to get their food and napped the rest of the time. Indeed, one recent study showed that the average African hunter-gatherer burned fewer calories than the average London office worker. But the key was the hunter-gatherer also ate less. It seems that, like every other animal on the planet, in our natural state we eat exactly as many calories as we require for the exercise level we take on. Exercise more and you'll eat more. Exercise less and less is what you'll eat. It's kind of like breathing. If you work out, you consume more oxygen, and if you don't you consume less. No one would be insane enough to suggest that our oxygen intake is related to obesity, but that's effectively what many were saying about our calorie intake.

If the sedentary nature of Western lifestyles was not the obesity factor – and neither, surely, were the fashions (can flared jeans make you fat?) or the language – then I reasoned it could only be the food itself. Perhaps there's something about Western food that interferes with our ability to recognise calories properly or use them efficiently.

It didn't take me long to find a significant volume of research suggesting that this 'something' was sugar. Until the early 1800s, the 'white gold' had been a rare, expensive and highly prized possession of the more well to do. Having rotten teeth was even once considered a status symbol because it meant you could obviously afford sugar. This caused wannabes to invest heavily in coal dust and tar (for smearing on the teeth, of course).

From the nineteenth century onwards, sugar became steadily cheaper and steadily added to more and more foods. It travelled with Western civilisation like a plague-infested rat, and was often the very first 'food' adopted by traditional inhabitants of any land it touched. We like sugar. We like it a lot. And we like any food that contains it more than any food that doesn't. This little economic truth wasn't lost on the people who desired to make money out of selling us food. All manner of new sugar-delivery vehicles were invented to tempt us – soft drinks were born in the dying days of the nineteenth century, chocolate bars at the start of the twentieth, and juices and sugar-filled breakfast cereals by the end of the 1940s.

But the science was abundantly clear by the mid-1950s. Sugar makes us fat. And not just us; any animal fed sugar will become obese, chronically ill and eventually die a horrible and gruesome death. Sugar isn't a poison in the sense that you drop dead on the spot, but it's a slow-acting poison that takes out your internal organs one by one – oh, and it makes you fat too. It seemed that the difference between animals that controlled their weight automatically and those that couldn't was the absence or presence of sugar.

The science about this was clear in the middle of last century. It's true that many i's had to be dotted and t's crossed to make the case bulletproof, but even then it was looking strong. By the time I was reading about it in the early 21st century, the detailed human trials had been done. We knew exactly how sugar destroys our bodies and exactly what biochemical pathways it uses. This was news to me. I had struggled my whole life with weight and appetite, and was probably on the path to an early grave or an unpleasant, lingering, drug-assisted old age because of something science had known about for a good half-century. I was a bit miffed. It seems the reason I'd never heard that news was there was too much money between me and the science. The science could have been yelling at me from my office door but I still wouldn't have heard it through the 6-feet-thick wall of food-industry money between me and the message.

The food industry's purpose is to make money. It's not there to make me healthy. It's there to sell me more stuff. If selling me sugar moves more product and doesn't kill me instantly, then the food industry will make more money. It's therefore in its best interests to ensure that nothing that could interfere with its ability to include as much sugar as it wishes ever sees the light of day. And so, just as tobacco companies did, the food industry suppresses, obfuscates and confuses any science that might suggest sugar is dangerous.

But my blinkers had been removed. I had read the science and (eventually) understood it. There was no doubt that the source of my weight problem was sugar. So I stopped eating it.

Forty kilograms melted away (over eighteen months) without me changing anything else about my lifestyle. I didn't exercise more. I didn't stop eating meat pies (and still haven't). I ate cheese and cream (not together – well, all right, once). And without exercising any willpower I achieved the one thing that had eluded me all my life: control of my weight. Even more importantly, I felt immensely clearer in the head, immensely more capable. I was also immensely more help to Lizzie, who was trying to breastfeed twins and wrangle four other tiny tots simultaneously.

Deleting sugar works its weight-control magic by handing you back mastery of your appetite. You find yourself suddenly unable to finish meals you would have wolfed down before. And you find yourself, mindful that your body won't let you eat much, getting picky about exactly what you'll waste your calories on. If someone had offered me a free meal before I quit sugar, I would have leapt at it regardless of what it was or whether I'd just eaten. But suddenly I found myself thinking blasphemous thoughts about whether I really wanted fries with that. It was unheard of. I was actually making decisions about food rather than having it (and clever marketing) drive my decisions. I was eating to live rather than living to eat.

Once I had that clarity and distance from food, I kept reading. When I was looking for sugar evidence, I'd noticed some disturbing research about another modern ingredient but I'd pushed it aside because it didn't seem relevant to my primary motivation – weight loss. Now that mission had been accomplished I came back to the material on vegetable oils. Like sugar, they'd only very recently made their way into the human diet. Before the twentieth century, the only fats we'd used in our entire history as a species came from animals or warm-climate fruit (such as coconuts, olives and avocados). But as the world was slugging it out on the battlefields of Flanders during the First World War, the food industry was discovering there was a much cheaper way to make cooking fats: squeeze them out of virtually worthless seeds such as cottonseed and soybean.

Those fats could be made for a poofteenth of the cost of animal fats and (with the right engineering) could be made to behave like their more expensive cousins once they were incorporated into food. Once again, ingestion didn't seem to cause instant death, so it was full steam ahead for the profit-driven food companies (that would be all of them).

The research I'd noticed had been produced as a by-product of human trials to prove that margarine (made from seed oils) lowers heart disease risk. It doesn't and the trials proved it, but what they also seemed to show was significant increases in cancer risk for the margarine eaters. Those trials were completed in the 1970s, but the results once again never made it to the front page. There was too much money drowning out the science. But the science didn't stop. Since then it has linked the types of fats present in seed oils to cancer, macular degeneration, heart disease, arthritis, allergies and Parkinson's disease. There's even very worrying research linking them to our epidemics of autoimmune disorders such as multiple sclerosis and lupus. In other words, if the chronic diseases caused by sugar don't get you, the ones caused by seed oils almost certainly will. But unlike the sugar diseases, by the time you have symptoms of the vegetable oil diseases you're irreversibly damaged. That was enough for me to ban them in our house immediately (and luckily Lizzie let me).

This book is a guided tour of what I found out about how our food supply and health messages have been perverted to provide profit rather than health. But more importantly, it's also a practical guide to doing something about it. No, I don't mean chaining yourself to a Coke truck, I mean knowing what to buy, what to eat, and when you need to start from scratch and when you don't. That section could be very short if everybody had the time and the inclination to grow, harvest and cook everything they ate. But since we usually also have to fit in earning a living, subsistence agriculture is unlikely to be a viable alternative for most. So I've tried to show where it's safe to compromise for the sake of convenience and where you'll be taking risks if you do. I also have a weather eye on the budget. You won't find me advocating superfoods such as chia seeds, goji berries or dolphin sweat (yep, I made that up, don't try to buy it). Every recommendation in this book is based on stuff you'll find in your average supermarket. I know this because that's exactly where Lizzie and I shop. And I won't recommend you try anything we haven't tried ourselves.

This is a book about eating real food in a society designed to make sure you do anything but Eat Real Food.

Part One

WHY WE SHOULD EAT REAL FOOD

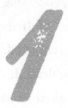

REAL FOOD VERSUS PROCESSED FOOD

What is processed food?

Let's start with some definitions. I'll frequently refer to something called *processed food*. What I mean by that is food manufactured in a factory. It's pretty easy to identify. It comes in a box, packet or bottle and it has a (usually long) list of ingredients. I reckon there are three categories of food:

1. **whole food:** something that until very recently was alive (or comes from something that is still alive) and has had almost nothing done to it other than kill it or pick it and place it on sale. These types of foods don't need labels and rarely have them. Any whole fruit or vegetable, nuts, grains, meat, milk and eggs are all whole foods.

2. **assembled food:** a mixture of whole foods that have had some minimal processing (the kind you could do at home if you wanted) applied to them. Butter is cream that has been churned. Cheese is the curd of milk that has been cultured. Bread is grains that have been crushed and baked. And olive oil is fruit that has been crushed and sieved.

3. **processed food:** looks like assembled food (or at least it does in the picture on the label), but is made in a factory using a multitude of ingredients, most of which would not be recognisable to the average punter. Margarine is fake butter, low-fat anything is a fake version of what it purports to be and anything liquid that didn't come from a mammal (such as a cow) or a tap is processed food.

For the entirety of our history as a species, except the last 200 years, we have eaten exclusively from the first two categories. Before the nineteenth century we simply didn't have the capacity to make, transport or store imitation food. Food usually had to be killed or picked and eaten within days. And even assembled food had a very limited shelf life. Refrigeration would not be available to most people until after the Second World War. It's not that our forebears objected to margarine or frozen pizza on philosophical or scientific grounds, they just didn't have a choice.

What is real food?

Real food is anything from the first two categories listed above. It's the whole food that has exclusively sustained us for all but the last 10,000 years (for the first 23 hours of my 24-hour clock). And it's the assembled food that enabled us to switch from hunting and gathering to town-based life (and that fed us all for the next 57 minutes of the 24-hour clock). In other words, it's everything but the processed food that now dominates the modern supermarket.

But this doesn't mean you need to start knitting your own underwear, haunting farmers' markets, being on first-name terms with the staff at the local biodynamic health-food store, keeping chooks, milking cows and breeding your own yeast (unless you want to). Real food is also still available in the average supermarket; you just have to walk past a lot of food-like substances to get to it.

Real food lurks on the fringes of the supermarket. It's the stuff you find in the fruit and vegetables section, the meat cabinet, the dairy section and the bread aisle. Not everything you find there is real food – there's still plenty of low-fat yoghurt; hi-fibre, low-GI bread; and light milk – but in those sections, it's the real food that dominates.

A short way of saying this is that if your great-grandparents were transported by a time machine from the early twentieth century to your local supermarket, the things they could identify as food would be the things you should load into your trolley (with the possible exception of chocolates and soft drinks).

**Real food is the food of our great-grandparents.
It's the food on the perimeter of the
supermarket. Everything else is slightly less
good for you than the box it's packed in.**

By now you may have spotted the catch in all this 'just eat real food' stuff. That's right, some assembly will be required. Cooking a roast dinner will involve more than opening the packet and setting the microwave to 'stun'. You'll need to know what temperature to put the oven on, you'll need to know how long to leave the roast in the oven. You'll need to know how to steam a vegetable (and for how long) and you'll probably want to know how to make gravy. All of that is a bit of a time-consuming bother when there's a perfectly similar (-looking) alternative available from a packet in just seconds. But the science tells us it's a bother well and truly worth having.

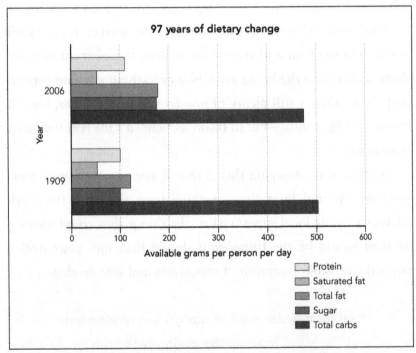

An adult in the United States eats about the same amount of protein and saturated fat as they did in 1909. They eat less non-sugar carbs but a lot more sugar and a lot more polyunsaturated fat.

Obviously there are differences between what we eat now and what Ned Kelly ate. I don't ever recall seeing a picture of Ned chugging an Up&Go breakfast drink before taking on the Victorian police, for example. But strip away two centuries of marketing gloss and some pretty fancy preservatives, and you find just two significant differences between 21st-century food and nineteenth-century food. Two hundred years ago, humans ate approximately what they'd been eating for the 10,000 (or in some cases 250,000) years before that. Where they lived (and how much money they had) affected the exact mix, but in general their diet was a mixture of vegetables, legumes and nuts, grains, meat, fish and an occasional fruit.

Some people had diets high in grains – for example, the British (barley and wheat) and the Japanese (rice); some people had diets high in vegetables – for example, the Indians (from India); some people had diets high in vegetable carbohydrates – for example, Polynesians (taro); some people had diets high in fat – for example, the Inuit (Eskimos); and some people had diets high in offal (the Americans and Australians). The proportions of carbohydrate (from grains), protein (from meat) and fat (from meat and fruit) varied enormously. But at the biochemical level, they all had one thing in common: none of these traditional diets contained significant quantities of sugar or polyunsaturated fats.

The following chapters set out a potted history of those two ingredients. I explain what they are and how we came to be eating so much of them. But most importantly I outline the science (not too much, I promise) on why that matters. These two ingredients are singlehandedly responsible for 90 per cent or more of the chronic disease that now plagues us in the West. Read on to find out how.

SUGAR

In the early nineteenth century, the average adult American (and Australian) was eating less than three teaspoons (12.6 grams) of added sugar (not counting the sugar in fruit and the lactose in milk) a day. One century later that number had increased

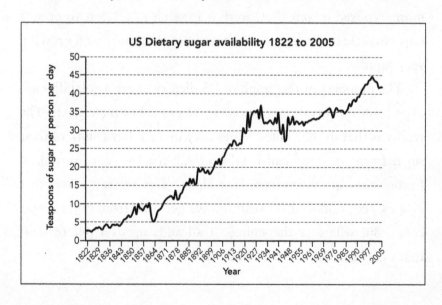

by a factor of ten, to 27 teaspoons (113 grams) a day. Roll forward another century and we are gobbling down more than 40 teaspoons (168 grams) a day.

You can draw a graph like the one above for any country exposed to a Western diet. The only thing that changes is the date the curve starts going upwards. That's the date when the traditional diet was replaced. In Australia, the United States and the United Kingdom, we started supplementing our traditional diet with serious amounts of sugar in the early 1800s, but in India it didn't start happening until they started importing our diet after the Second World War. As late as 1963, the average Indian was consuming just three teaspoons of sugar a day (10 per cent of our consumption then). But now they are catching up to us quickly, with a fivefold increase in consumption since then. China was even later to the party. In 1978 the average rural Chinese was consuming just 730 grams of sugar a year (less than half a teaspoon a day). Even their city cousins, who were more exposed to our diet, were managing just 1.5 teaspoons a day. Now their consumption is ten times that much and growing very rapidly.

The numbers in the graph of US dietary sugar availability are expressed in equivalent teaspoons (4.2 grams) of table sugar. The reality is that in the United States they make a fair chunk of their sugar from corn and call it HFCS (high-fructose corn syrup), in Europe they get theirs from beet plants (yep, the same ones that give us beetroot) and in Australia we get ours from grass (sugar cane). But whatever the source, it all adds up to a pile of stuff that's half glucose and half fructose.

THE DEFINITION OF SUGAR?

Sugar is the white stuff you put in your tea. A chemist would call it sucrose. And that same chemist (or a different one, your choice) would tell you sucrose is a molecule of glucose joined to a molecule of fructose.

Our body doesn't care if the packet of sugar says it's brown sugar, caster sugar, raw sugar, even low-GI sugar, all it sees is sucrose. And by the time they hit our bloodstream they are all just glucose and fructose.

Glucose is our fuel supply. Every cell in our body uses glucose to produce energy. Every carbohydrate (foods made from grains, milk, fruit, vegetables, nuts and legumes) we eat is converted into glucose and supplied to our cells for energy.

Fructose cannot be used by our body for energy. We are poorly adapted to it because, before the invention of sugar, we only encountered it in ripe fruit (when in season) or (if we were very lucky) in honey. We don't waste it, though. Our liver very efficiently converts fructose into stored energy (largely fat).

Today in Australia almost all the sugar we encounter in processed food is sucrose. All that sucrose massively increases our exposure to the once relatively rare fructose.

We make our sugar from grass (cane sugar) but it has the same amount of fructose even if it's made from corn (high-fructose corn syrup favoured by the Americans) or beet plants (beet sugar favoured by the Europeans) or fruit (fruit juice concentrate favoured by processed food manufacturers who want to say 'No added cane sugar' on the label).

Why did sugar consumption increase so much?

We haven't always had access to loads of sugar. Before the nineteenth century, sugar was a luxury reserved for the very well heeled. It was so expensive that people who could afford it would display it proudly on their dinner table in ornate silver 'sugar boxes'. The only sugar most ordinary people could access was in the form of fresh fruit or honey (if they were lucky enough to live somewhere where either was available).

Throughout the early 1800s, the price of sugar had been steadily falling as newer and more reliable methods of farming and extracting it were invented. But in the 1830s, sugar-production technology leapt forward in the United States. Steam-driven mills drove the price of white gold ever lower, and it was increasingly used by more and more food manufacturers and householders alike. We really like sugar, and when it's cheap enough we like it even more. For the first time in human history, sugar became a common food ingredient in the average person's diet.

At the start of the nineteenth century, the average American was eating just a couple of teaspoons of sugar a day. By the start of the twentieth century that had increased by a factor of ten. A whole new food category, the sugar hit, had been invented, and we had recipes for sweet treats coming out our ears. Sugar was a cheap, desirable way to feed the masses. We had jams, tarts, pastries, boiled lollies, cakes, jellies and, by the start of the new century, chocolate bars and sugar water. Cadbury discovered that adding sugar to the bitter condiment cocoa made magic happen (especially to their bottom line), and entrepreneurs in the United States had discovered that dumping a load of sugar in carbonated water made even more magic happen.

By the 1950s, American sugar intake had almost doubled again. Even though sugar rationing during the Second World War had seriously impacted availability, two inventions ensured sugar stayed a significant part of our diet after the war. Household refrigeration was becoming a must-have, and it meant that we could have sugar–water and fruit juice on hand all the time. But the real kicker was the brilliant idea to add massive amounts of sugar to breakfast cereals. Until then, eating cereal for breakfast was really only something done by vegetarians or people with a need to unclog the pipes (so to speak). The advent of the sugary children's cereal saw breakfast cereal sales double every nine years during the mid-twentieth century.

Food manufacturers knew that food with sugar sells a lot better than food without sugar, so they made sure their brand always had more sugar than the brands next to it on the supermarket shelves. Sugar increases sales, so it's embedded in everything and our total consumption grows ever higher.

The fourteen ways sugar messes with your body

It's the fructose half of that massive increase in sugar that wreaks havoc on our body. Never before in our history as a species have we been exposed to more than two teaspoons of sugar's worth of fructose a day. The twentyfold increase in the last two centuries is increasingly being nailed by science as the primary cause of most of the chronic diseases that currently afflict us. In the pages that follow I give a quick tour of the science that backs up a statement like that. This is a long book so this is necessarily a Cook's tour. If you want the detail on the science of the damage done by sugar then I recommend you take a look at my first book, *Sweet Poison*. If, however, you're someone who just likes skipping to the end of a book to see whodunnit, then here's the list.

The fourteen ways fructose will destroy your body

1. Fructose rots your teeth.
2. Fructose inflames your gut.
3. Fructose destroys your liver.
4. Fructose takes out your pancreas (and your eyes and limbs).
5. Fructose makes you fat.
6. Fructose messes up your kidneys.
7. Fructose gives you gout.
8. Fructose creates high blood pressure (hypertension).
9. Fructose destroys erectile function.
10. Fructose makes women infertile.
11. Fructose takes out your heart.
12. Fructose destroys your brain.
13. Fructose makes you depressed (and anxious).
14. Fructose feeds cancer.

In short, there are two primary disease trajectories caused by fructose. One is the series of diseases caused by it being immediately converted to fat by our liver. That little trigger cascades into fatty liver disease, type 2 diabetes, polycystic ovary syndrome (PCOS), obesity, heart disease and Alzheimer's disease. The other is the group of diseases that originate in uric acid being produced as part of that fat-creation process. This produces the gout, erectile dysfunction, hypertension and kidney disease. But let's start at the point of entry – your teeth.

1 Fructose rots your teeth

Your teeth are the first part of your body to touch fructose and, like the proverbial canary in the coalmine, they are usually the first to suffer its effects. The numbers don't lie. Populations exposed to sugar for the first time go from 'background' levels of tooth decay (around four cavities per 100 teeth) to 'modern' levels (around 24 cavities per 100 teeth). The mechanism has been known since the 1960s and the science is uncontroversial.

We also know why sugar affects our teeth this way. Normally when we eat anything, bacteria in our mouth also get a meal. As they chomp down on our lunch they produce acid waste that, if left in contact with our teeth, can destroy the protective enamel coating. But we didn't come down in the last shower. Our saliva neutralises the acid and flushes out the mouth within twenty minutes of eating – no harm, no foul and especially no decay. This is why human populations that aren't exposed to Western food have barely any tooth decay.

It's a beautiful system. Unfortunately, fructose completely stuffs it up. If what we eat includes the fructose half of sugar then the bacteria can use it to create a defensive shield against saliva. This shield, called plaque, holds the acid against the tooth surface and stops saliva washing it away. I reckon I'd be pushed to think of a better way to destroy tooth enamel, the hardest substance in the human body. Fructose is the magic ingredient that turns largely harmless mouth bacteria into teeth-eroding monsters.

2 Fructose inflames your gut

Our small intestine works by being permeable only to stuff we can use (like food) and impermeable to anything that might potentially hurt us (like bacteria). But when we consume some substances, our gut becomes permeable, and toxic molecules normally attached to bacteria (endotoxins) escape through our intestinal walls and into our bloodstream. Our immune system has an inflammation reaction to endotoxins, and this response causes our gut to become inflamed. The increasingly prevalent irritable bowel syndrome (IBS) is likely to be simply a warning that our body is trying hard to deal with that increased gut permeability.

Binge drinking alcohol will produce exactly that effect, but so too will overconsumption of fructose. If you drink alcohol all day every day, then any fructose you consume won't add noticeably to the problem. But if you're like most people and your hourly poison of choice is sugar, then it, rather than booze, is probably responsible for your inflamed gut.

Unfortunately, both alcohol and fructose also appear to increase the populations of bacteria that produce endotoxins in our small intestine (something charmingly termed bacterial overgrowth). So we get the double whammy of more endotoxins in our gut and doors left ajar (gut permeability) to let them into our bloodstream.

It's early days yet but the science is also increasingly showing that bacterial overgrowth (caused by fructose consumption) is likely to be the cause of the massive increase in stomach acid reflux disorders, such as heartburn and gastro-oesophageal reflux disease (GORD).

3 Fructose destroys your liver

We're adapted to a diet where most carbohydrates are glucose or glucose-based. Almost all the glucose we consume is diverted to the parts of our body that need it most, largely our muscles and brain. It's our primary fuel. If we were cars, glucose would be what we'd be pumping into the tank every half-price Tuesday. So we have exquisitely finely tuned feedback loops that tell us we're full when we've taken on enough glucose.

Those loops don't fire for fructose. Our body doesn't recognise it as fuel. It's like filling your car with diesel instead of unleaded. So after fructose hits your bloodstream, it's ignored by all the cells needing fuel and the next stop is the liver. Our body is a little smarter than the car – we can filter out the incorrect fuel and store it in case we need it later. Our liver can make fructose useful by converting it into fat, so that's exactly what it does. That fat is stored in the liver, and some of it is exported into our bloodstream as molecules called triglycerides (three [tri-] fat molecules attached to a sugar [glyceride] backbone).

The stored fat builds and builds until the liver becomes bloated with fat. That condition is called non-alcoholic fatty liver disease, or just fatty liver. Because our diet is now so high in fructose, one in three adult Australians has fatty liver and the number is increasing rapidly. That is 1000 times the number that have its cousin, alcoholic fatty liver disease (caused by, well, see if you can guess). Fatty liver usually has no symptoms until it's well advanced, and most cases are discovered accidentally when liver tests are being done for other reasons. But left untreated, fatty liver can progress through various disease stages and ultimately end in cirrhosis requiring a liver transplant. There is now interesting scientific speculation that the trigger for converting mere fatty liver into cirrhosis is our immune response to endotoxins leaking from the gut because of fructose consumption. So fructose delivers twice – it opens the gut and fattens the liver, the two things we need to ensure our liver is destroyed by cirrhosis.

4 Fructose takes out your pancreas (and your eyes and limbs)

Our bodies convert most carbohydrates to glucose. In healthy people that glucose is pumped out via our bloodstream to the cells that require energy, bringing blood-glucose levels down quickly after a meal. These cells signal their need for glucose by moving insulin receptors to the cell surface (kinda like hanging out the 'this room needs servicing' sign in a hotel). When insulin in the blood (which is released by our pancreas in response to high blood-glucose levels) meets these receptors, the cell opens its glucose 'gates' and lets in exactly as much glucose as it requires. But when fructose-derived fat accumulates in the liver and bloodstream, it affects something called insulin sensitivity. The insulin receptors never get to the cell surface (or if they do, it's in smaller numbers). The result is that the glucose goes sailing by. The sign never gets put on the door handle and the room doesn't get serviced. Our bodies starve in a sea of food.

Because the glucose doesn't get used by the cells, it stays in the bloodstream longer and the result is a high blood-sugar concentration for longer than normal. This is called insulin resistance or pre-diabetes. Our body usually responds to insulin resistance by pumping up the insulin levels until the glucose is cleared. For most of us, if we ask our body to run on overdrive like that for years, our pancreas (the insulin maker) will pack it in. Then we'll need daily insulin injections to live. Along the way, the persistently high blood glucose will result in blindness and limb amputations for many sufferers.

5 Fructose makes you fat

What we think of as our 'appetite' is really just the tangible readout from our energy-management system. When we need energy, our appetite increases and we seek out fuel (food to you and me). When we've taken enough fuel on board, our appetite shuts down and makes us feel stuffed so we don't eat any more. The hormones that tell us we've had enough are triggered by the amount of food entering our bloodstream, cholecystokinin (CCK) for fat and insulin for carbohydrates. Unfortunately, one food doesn't trigger the release of either of these primary appetite-control hormones. Can you guess what it might be? That's right, fructose. It's completely ignored by the system that's supposed to tell us to stop eating. This means the energy from fructose is not being counted at all by our bodies. But far worse than just being ignored, fructose actively messes up our ability to tell how much food we really need.

The fructose half of sugar is an appetite-hormone disruptor. With sugar in our diet, our bodies can no longer tell when we've had enough food. It's as if our appetite-control system is stuck at half-off. Sugar gives our bodies permission to keep on eating, and

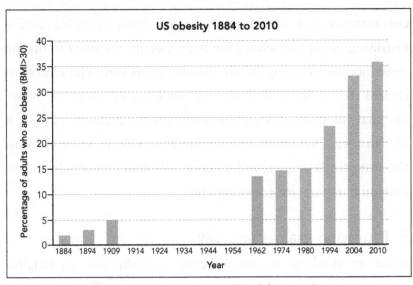

US obesity 1884 to 2010

In 1884 less than one in every 50 adults was obese.
Now more than one in three is.
Note: No surveys were taken between 1909 and 1962.

we don't stop until we're physically restrained by the size of our stomach (or jeans). When that problem, well, passes, our broken appetite control gives us permission to keep eating until we're stuffed again. The result is that we're eating way too much, and our hormones, fabulous as they are, can't read a calorie sticker slapped on a board at KFC so we just keep on eating. This is why, in the United States for example, the average daily food intake has increased by 30 per cent in the last three decades.

Insulin tells us we've had enough to eat, which is great as long as we can hear it. But when fructose causes us to become insulin resistant (see point 4 above), we don't get the message and our fuel-management system can veer wildly out of control. A disrupted appetite-control system will store too much fuel. We have loads but we can't use it because of the insulin resistance, so it circulates in our bloodstream. But we have a plan B. When the pancreas attempts to cope with elevated blood glucose (caused by fructose-derived fat) by ramping up insulin, it's only fixing the immediate problem. All that extra insulin doesn't make the damaged cells any less insulin resistant, it just means that undamaged cells use the insulin to make fat. In other words the blood glucose is cleared from the bloodstream by making us fatter. Obesity is a symptom of the failure in the balance of hormones controlling how much food we take in.

Just for good measure, fructose also interferes directly with leptin signalling. Leptin is our long-term energy-storage hormone. It's produced by fat cells and tells us not to eat between meals. The way it's supposed to work is that the more fat cells we have, the more leptin we produce and the less we eat. Unfortunately, fructose makes us less sensitive to that hormone as well, so we eat more of everything, not just more sugar.

This fructose-induced double dose of hormone dysfunction causes us to store too much fat in our cells, but our body isn't aware the fat is there and keeps demanding food. Our appetite-control system thinks we're starving even while we have more than enough fat being packed away (usually in very unsightly places). It's like having a car with a busted fuel gauge. It constantly says the tank is empty even if it's full. Except this car will let you keep on putting more fuel in, and the fructose eater will keep gaining weight.

6 Fructose messes up your kidneys

When fructose is converted to fat by our liver, a significant amount of a waste product called uric acid is produced. But we're well adapted to deal with it, because it's also produced when we eat meat and drink alcohol. Our kidneys are our built-in pool filter for removing waste products like uric acid. But they can be overwhelmed by the quantities produced by the fructose levels in a modern Western diet. When that happens, our kidneys start to fail. And this is likely to be why excess uric acid has been associated with significant increases in kidney disease in a long line of rat studies and more recently in human trials.

The number of us requiring treatment for kidney disease has nearly doubled in the last decade. It's now killing more Australians than either breast or prostate cancer, and is responsible for one in every seven hospitalisations in this country. It's massively destructive to our quality of life and ultimately lethal for far too many of us. But the saddest part is that most of the horror of this epidemic is preventable just by eliminating fructose from the diet.

7 Fructose gives you gout

Unlike many of the other conditions in this list, gout won't kill you. But its presence is very definitely an early warning sign for the kidney disease that can. Gout is an acute inflammatory arthritis usually affecting the big toe, but it can also strike heels, knees, wrists and fingers. It's caused by high levels of uric acid accumulating in the blood and then crystallising in the joints. Our immune system reacts to the foreign substance in the joint, and this causes the pain and inflammation.

Gout was once a rare disease strongly associated with wealth, so much so that it was dubbed the 'disease of kings' because it was known to be caused by excessive eating and drinking. But it's now very much a disease of the everyman. And I say 'man' quite intentionally there. Most gout sufferers are men in their forties, although increasingly, postmenopausal women are among those affected. As with many other conditions caused by fructose, it seems that being of child-bearing age affords some temporary protection. But it's very much a disease on the march. Fructose has now become the primary uric acid generator for most of us, and a recent British study found that the number of people affected had increased by 64 per cent in just fifteen years, and the number of women affected had doubled. One in 40 Britons now has gout, and there's no reason to believe that Australia's statistics are any less frightening.

Of course, this means that since gout and kidney failure are caused by the same overabundance of uric acid, if you suffer from gout you should get your kidney function tested. But wait, there's more. From the very moment it was first described in 1879, high blood pressure has been linked to gout and the level of uric acid in the bloodstream.

8 Fructose creates high blood pressure (hypertension)

Trial after trial conducted between 1972 and 2005 has shown that we're twice as likely to suffer from hypertension if we have high uric acid levels. Uric acid deactivates nitric oxide, a muscle relaxant that keeps the smooth muscle cells of our artery walls dilated, so when uric acid levels are high, the artery walls become more rigid. This reduces the diameter of our arteries, which increases our blood pressure (as any plumber will tell you, a thinner pipe means higher pressure). Recent human studies have conclusively demonstrated that to give healthy volunteers hypertension, all you need do is feed them fructose.

The reason for all the interest is that there are drugs (drug companies have much deeper pockets for this kind of research) that can be used to lower uric acid levels. Recent human trials have shown that these drugs do indeed lower blood pressure, but the evidence is clear that there's a much simpler preventative measure for all the conditions related to uric acid – kidney disease, gout and hypertension. Don't eat or drink sugar.

WHAT ABOUT SALT?

We've been told for a long time that salt causes high blood pressure. But when that hypothesis has been put to the test the results have been all over the map. Sometimes it does, sometimes it doesn't and sometimes it actually lowers it. And even when salt reduction does show an improvement, the effect is about the same as you might expect if the person was asked to drink less water before the test (about a 2 per cent improvement). Fructose (delivered in the form of just one 700 ml soft drink per day), on the other hand, definitively increases blood pressure by 5–10 per cent. If blood pressure is a problem for you, then the research says the white crystal you should be worrying about is more likely to be found in the sugar bowl than the salt shaker.

9 Fructose destroys erectile function

Around one in five US men now suffers from erectile dysfunction. But one of the more recent studies tells us that one in two men with type 2 diabetes will suffer the problem.

We know exactly what causes most of it – a lack of nitric oxide, the same beastie that prevents high blood pressure (see point 8). When its production is suppressed, erectile function becomes seriously impaired because the blood simply can't get through. Viagra, Levitra and Cialis work by temporarily encouraging the production of nitric oxide.

We know that the opposite of Viagra is uric acid. Uric acid produced as a result of fructose consumption reacts dramatically with our homegrown nitric oxide, thereby effectively deactivating it. If we have large amounts of uric acid in our bloodstream, we can expect our nitric oxide to be rendered ineffective. No effective nitric oxide means no erectile function.

It should also then come as no particular surprise that erectile dysfunction is closely aligned with the other symptoms of overindulging in fructose, namely heart disease, obesity and type 2 diabetes, and that the number of men needing assistance is increasing as rapidly as the incidence of those diseases.

Perhaps if sugar were renamed anti-Viagra, people might think twice about consuming it.

10 Fructose makes women infertile

Polycystic ovary syndrome (PCOS) is the primary cause of female infertility in Australia today. As many as one in six Australian women of reproductive age now has PCOS. The symptoms usually include acne, the appearance of male patterns of hair growth (and male-pattern baldness) and irregular or absent periods. Okay, so it's not pleasant, but the big impact is on fertility. A recent Swedish evaluation concluded that women with PCOS were nine times more likely to need access to IVF than women without the syndrome. IVF is the last resort in fertility treatment. It's used when everything else has failed. And it's being used increasingly frequently. The number of IVF treatments grew by 50 per cent between 2004 and 2009 and is currently increasing by about 14 per cent every year. In Australia today, approximately one in every 30 children is born as a result of IVF. And given that IVF is often unsuccessful, those numbers are a significant understatement of the number of people using the treatment.

As you might expect from a glance at the symptoms, PCOS is a result of too much testosterone (the male sex hormone). Testosterone is not an exclusively male hormone. Women have it too, but generally at about 10 per cent of the male level. Doctors have long known that women with PCOS have not only higher testosterone levels, but also extremely low levels of a very important protein, the charmingly named sex hormone binding globulin (SHBG). By binding to testosterone, SHBG controls the amount of free (and therefore active) testosterone in our bloodstream. Low levels of SHBG in women seem to result in too much free testosterone.

It's also well established that people who are obese or have insulin resistance or type 2 diabetes have extremely low levels of SHBG. Hormones are complex things (and that's an understatement) and sex hormones are the big daddy of complexity. Because they're constantly produced and their actions depend on the presence or absence of other sex hormones and our gender, it's very hard to tease out the cause and the effect. For a long time researchers have believed that insulin resistance caused low SHBG. That would mean that PCOS was a consequence of being insulin resistant. But a recent study has shown this isn't the case. It turns out that insulin levels don't affect the level of SHBG, but the presence of fat around the liver affects both insulin and SHBG levels. And we already know that fatty liver is a direct consequence of eating fructose.

So it looks like insulin resistance, type 2 diabetes, fatty liver disease and PCOS are all part of the same bunch of joy you can expect from consuming fructose. And in any event, it's clear from the research that fructose directly increases the amount of circulating testosterone in women (by depressing SHBG). More testosterone directly impairs a woman's ability to conceive. The single most effective way for a woman with PCOS to increase her chances of having a baby is to stop eating fructose.

11 Fructose takes out your heart

Throughout this chapter I've referred to heart disease. By that I mean all the diseases caused by atherosclerosis (hardening of the arteries). This group includes myocardial infarction (what most people call a heart attack), ischemic stroke and arterial thrombosis (the blocking of arteries in the limbs). Atherosclerosis affects all arteries but is most common in the big ones transporting the highest volumes of blood, such as those near the heart and brain.

Some of the fat generated by fructose in the liver stays there, but the rest is exported into the bloodstream. Because fat isn't soluble in a water-based solution like blood, it's transported by specialised proteins called lipoproteins (*lipo* is Greek for 'fat'). Lipoproteins come in a variety of sizes according to how much fat they can carry. There are various types, ranging from low-density lipoprotein (LDL cholesterol, often called 'bad cholesterol') to high-density lipoprotein (HDL cholesterol, often called 'good cholesterol'). Within each of these categories is a range of sizes and densities, and scientists are now certain that having lots of larger, fluffier LDL particles puts us in the lowest risk category for heart disease. People like that are called pattern A. People who have lots of smaller and less fluffy LDL particles are called pattern B and are the most likely to suffer a heart attack.

Fructose is exported from the liver in small dense LDL particles. The most efficient way to convert someone from pattern A (safe) to pattern B (at risk) is to feed them fructose. The second best way is to put them on a diet low in saturated fat. We use lipoproteins to transport the fat we eat as well as the fat we make from fructose. We know now that a diet high in saturated fat will produce pattern A LDL particles. In other words, eating saturated fat lowers your risk of heart disease. So it seems the best way to ensure you're a candidate for heart disease is to eat sugar or avoid saturated fat or, as many now do, both. Cholesterol (mostly manufactured by the liver – the quantity we eat is infinitesimally tiny compared to the amount we make) is also transported in the lipoproteins, but its job in our body is repairing damage. Yes, cholesterol is always on the scene at the arterial lesions that cause heart disease, but that's because it's doing its job. Blaming cholesterol for heart disease is like blaming ambulance drivers for car accidents just because you notice they always seem to be there when an accident occurs.

In short, then, cholesterol doesn't cause heart disease but a high-sugar, low-fat diet does. If you're thinking this is the opposite of what we've been told for the last 50 years, you're right. If you want to know why we've been told that and how terribly wrong researchers have been with their advice, then take a look at my detailed history of fat and cholesterol research in *Big Fat Lies*.

12 Fructose destroys your mind

Many researchers are now referring to Alzheimer's (the most common form of dementia) as type 3 diabetes. As for type 2 diabetes (see point 4), long-term insulin resistance and high blood sugar are common symptoms for Alzheimer's sufferers. So it seems fructose can either destroy your brain with an acute event like a stroke (see point 11) or take a more leisurely approach and destroy your mind first with dementia.

A series of recent studies have confirmed that we are two to four times more likely to suffer from dementia if we have type 2 diabetes and that the longer we've been insulin resistant the higher the probability.

One of the recent studies (which used precise cognitive testing) was even able to put an exact number on it, finding that each 1 per cent rise in long-term average blood sugar takes us two whole years closer to dementia.

Persistently high blood sugar is caused by insulin resistance, which in turn is caused by overconsumption of fructose. And the research clearly suggests that the next step in that deadly cascade is dementia. If you're interested in exactly how fructose forms the plaques that are characteristic of Alzheimer's, then take a look at the section on AGEs (advanced glycation end products) in *Big Fat Lies*.

13 Fructose makes you depressed (and anxious)

We can become depressed because things aren't going well. If having your cat run over doesn't alter your mood (one way or the other depending on how you feel about cats, I guess) then you were probably built by aliens. But the science suggests that how long we stay depressed has more to do with biochemistry than Fluffy's road-safety skills.

Food makes us happy (shocking, I know). Even seeing food improves our mood. This is because the anticipation of a feed fires up the hormones responsible for how we feel. The sight (or smell) of food gives us a squirt of the pleasure hormone, dopamine. Dopamine focuses our attention, makes us think more clearly and helps us move faster and more effectively. It's an important signal to our body that we're in for something good and we need to pay attention. And that was probably pretty handy in times gone by. If you had to chase your food, being sharper was definitely an advantage.

Once we actually start eating, another hormone – serotonin – kicks in. Serotonin is the yin to dopamine's yang. It's our 'chill out, all's good' hormone. The serotonin makes us feel happier and less stressed. We relax, our mood improves (Fluffy will still be roadkill, but we'll feel better about it) and our minds can turn to less important things than eating. Sex, another thing important for keeping humans around, has exactly the same effect. Anticipation produces dopamine and 'achievement' produces serotonin.

Researchers have known for a long time that severe depression is strongly associated with an inability to absorb serotonin properly in the brain. No (or low) serotonin absorption makes it much harder for us to bounce back from unhappiness. And this can translate into anxiety and depression if it's sustained for long enough. The primary antidepressant drugs available in Australia (Cipramil, Luvox, Prozac, Lovan, Aropax and Zoloft) all work by targeting the serotonin system and giving the brain more time to absorb the serotonin. Some other drugs (ecstasy, amphetamines and LSD) work by enhancing the amount of serotonin we produce (but you might find it tricky to get a prescription for them).

If all is well with our hormone system, severe depression should be an extremely rare disease. But it's not. Depression is a major chronic health problem and it is getting much worse at a very rapid rate. Something is messing with our serotonin system and the evidence is starting to mount that the something is fructose. Fructose is the only carbohydrate that produces a significant spike in our cortisol levels. Cortisol is our stress hormone. It's terribly handy for confrontations with unexpected bears (for example) because it ramps up dopamine (to focus our mind and sharpen our movements). It also rapidly increases the amount of dopamine we can absorb. But it does so at the expense of our ability to absorb serotonin.

We like dopamine. It's our reward drug. It tells us we're about to get good stuff (like food and sex). Frequent hits of fructose mean frequent hits of dopamine. This leads inevitably to fructose addiction, and that's exactly the mechanism used by other man-made opioid drugs (such as nicotine and cocaine). The trouble is that it seems the up-regulation of dopamine at the expense of serotonin can become hardwired if we allow it to go on for long enough. And once we're addicted, we can't help but let it go on for long enough.

We don't run into that many bears on a daily basis (well, I don't). Fructose was once about as common as a bear encounter, but it's now embedded in almost every processed food we buy. And it has an addictive quality as powerful as that of nicotine. We're now on a constant drip of fructose. That means we're on a constant cortisol (and therefore dopamine) high. This in turn continuously impairs our ability to absorb serotonin, the one substance that can turn our mood around. Fluffy will still become a bumper sticker if he chooses an inopportune moment to cross the freeway, and that will probably be a downer. But the science is suggesting that how quickly (or if) we bounce back from that may depend on how much fructose we eat.

14 Fructose feeds cancer

Except in the case of organs directly affected by fructose (the liver, pancreas and kidneys), it's unlikely to cause cancer. For that we need to look at seed oils (see Chapter 3). But new research suggests that having fructose in the bloodstream will accelerate tumour growth.

We grow new cells all the time (particularly in the skin and gut) and we do so using cell division and reproduction. We aren't quite as good at it as some species of gecko that can grow back entire limbs, but we get by. If that cell reproduction gets out of control, because of a bug (say, a virus or something else that causes damage) in the DNA-controlling the process, then the cells would be unable to stop reproducing. We call this unchecked reproduction cancer. And we usually label it by the organ it's happening in or near (for example, skin cancer, liver cancer, etc.).

It's well established that consistently high blood-glucose levels (such as those suffered by a type 2 diabetic) will accelerate the growth of cancerous cells. A recent study from the University of California (UCLA) exposed human pancreatic cancer cells to solutions of pure glucose and pure fructose in the lab. The researchers knew both sugars would feed the cancer, but in this study they were trying to determine whether fructose had a more direct involvement in cancer growth. To find out, they tagged the sugars with radioactive carbon (so they could work out what the cells were doing with the sugars by seeing where the carbon ended up). They found that the fructose was metabolised very differently by the cancerous cells.

As expected, both halves of sugar (glucose and fructose) could be used for energy. But only fructose supplied significant quantities of the building materials for cancer growth. They found it was being used directly by the cells to maintain the much higher output of genetic material (DNA) that cells need in order to divide and proliferate. Cancer will occur whether we eat sugar or not (much more on the real causes in chapter three), but if we want to make sure that a cancer has the best possible chance of growing, then it looks like the best possible food we can consume is anything containing significant quantities of fructose.

Studies of cells in a lab setting are not overly persuasive on their own. There are a lot of checks and balances in a living organism that simply do not exist when you isolate one type of cell. For example, the cancer doesn't have to contend with an immune system trying to kill it. But these tests on pancreatic tumours combined with a strong line of population studies (coming to pretty much the same conclusion) are worth paying attention to.

The good news – it's all reversible

Obesity is a symptom of sugar consumption, but it's not the only one. Heart disease, type 2 diabetes, kidney disease and dementia, to name just a few, are all symptoms of the same underlying disorder. And, just as for any other disease, the same symptoms don't appear for everybody at the same time. Not all sufferers of kidney disease are obese, although most are. Not all victims of heart disease are obese, although most are. And 15 per cent of US (and probably a similar percentage of Australian) type 2 diabetes sufferers are not overweight. The good news with sugar is that the symptoms of almost all the conditions listed above are obvious. For most of us, the first sign will be gaining a few kilograms, but even without that signal, there will be early warning signs from some of the other conditions, such as your teeth falling out or hair growing where it shouldn't. While all of the conditions listed above will eventually result in permanent, irreparable damage (such as the removal of a kidney), before you get to that point the diseases are largely reversible.

All you need do is not eat fructose. As soon as you do that, all this badness goes into reverse. Your liver stops storing fructose-derived fat, your insulin sensitivity begins to reset, you start losing weight, your LDL particles switch back to pattern A, your nitric oxide levels increase and your gout disappears. Your body goes into repair mode once the Sweet Poison (I couldn't resist) is no longer a part of what you eat. Unfortunately, that's not the case for the set of diseases we're about to discuss. Disease states caused by polyunsaturated-fat consumption are largely permanent and sneak up on you much more silently. Even worse than that, unlike fructose, we can't taste the presence of polyunsaturated fat in our food, so we need to be extra, super vigilant. It's the original silent but deadly killer.

3

POLYUNSATURATED FAT

The changes in the types of fat we consume are much more recent but no less dramatic than the rapid increase in sugar consumption.

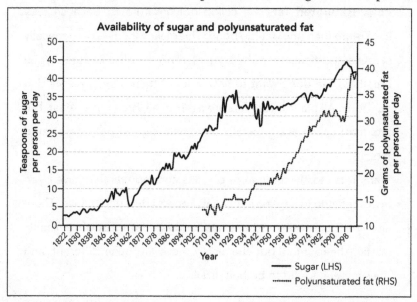

Availability of sugar and polyunsaturated fat

Sugar (LHS)
.... Polyunsaturated fat (RHS)

THE FOUR TYPES OF FAT

All fats consist mainly of a chain of carbon atoms with hydrogen atoms attached. Animals (including us) make fat from their food. The type we make is either saturated or monounsaturated.

Saturated fats are called saturated because every one of their carbon atoms is attached to four other atoms (one or two adjacent carbon atoms and two or more hydrogen atoms) by a single bond. In other words, their bonding capacity is saturated. This makes them unreactive, which is why they don't go rancid (react with oxygen).

Monounsaturated fats are called unsaturated because one of their carbon atoms is bonded to the adjacent carbon atom by a double bond, which means they can react more readily with other chemicals, such as oxygen.

But there's a type of fat we animals can't make. In addition to saturated and monounsaturated fats, plants can also make polyunsaturated fats.

Polyunsaturated fats are called polyunsaturated because they have more than one double bond. This makes them very chemically reactive (particularly with oxygen). This is why, being oxygen breathers, we don't want to have a lot of them running around in our body. All plant-based fats are a mix of all three types of fat, but fats from seeds are generally extremely high in polyunsaturated fats.

Trans fats mostly come from polyunsaturated fats that have been hydrogenated (using the industrial process I describe below). There also small quantities of trans fats found in the meat of ruminants (cattle, sheep, etc.), but chemically these are quite different, and they've been found to be beneficial.

At the start of the twentieth century, the average American adult consumed about 50 grams of saturated fat a day, a similar amount of monounsaturated fat (the two main fats in animal fat – see 'The four types of fat' on the opposite page) and 13 grams of polyunsaturated fat. These days, the average American adult consumes about the same amount of saturated fat, but 80 grams a day of monounsaturated fat and 40 grams a day of polyunsaturated fat. In one short century, we have tripled the amount of polyunsaturated fat in our diet and increased the amount of monounsaturated fat by more than half.

Why has polyunsaturated-fat consumption increased so much?

We eat polyunsaturated fat because it's cheap. Not cheap for us, but cheap for the people making the food we eat. As soon as we surrender control of assembly of our food, we also surrender control over the quality of the ingredients used. Over the last century this has meant that almost all the increasingly expensive animal fats humans had been successfully eating for the entire history of their presence on this planet were replaced by much cheaper fats manufactured from plant seeds.

In the early nineteenth century, the industrial revolution resulted in English farmers moving to cities in their millions. Families went to work in factories and stopped making their daily bread from scratch. The profession of baker came into its own, and the demand was incessant. It didn't take long before unscrupulous bakers discovered that many people couldn't tell if they padded out their (expensive but popular) wheat flour with some less edible substances such as alum (a poison used to whiten it), chalk, sawdust, and plaster of Paris. A similar thing was going on with used tea leaves bought from restaurants. They were recycled by being boiled in sheep dung and coloured with tannin before being resold. Because some of these things could be immediately lethal, chemists eventually raised the alarm and appropriate regulation was brought to bear.

But a similar thing has been going on with fat right under our noses for the last century, and not only have we not caught on, our health authorities are actively encouraging us to consume the processed food industry's equivalent of sawdust and dung.

The industrial revolution fuelled a population explosion that drove up the price of wheat (and therefore bread) and was also putting pressure on traditional sources of fat. Animal fat was becoming more expensive, so one chap who needed to buy a lot of it decided to do something. In 1869, Napoleon III offered a prize to anyone who could develop a cheap alternative to butter to feed to his troops. A chemist called Hippolyte Mège-Mouriès claimed the dosh by creating something passably edible out of lard (cheaper but still sourced from animals). His patented method was bought in 1871 by a Dutch company that is now part of Unilever, the maker of Flora margarine and loads of other stuff.

American inventors took the idea a step further by incorporating an even cheaper fat into the process. The US was under enormous population pressures. The number of Americans had doubled between 1880 and 1910 and all those extra mouths needed a cheap source of fat. The good news was it also had cottonseed waste coming out of its ears. And those cottonseeds were high in fat. Mixing cottonseed oil with the lard made it go an awful lot further and made the French fake butter even cheaper to manufacture.

But the new American fake-butter purveyors wanted to eliminate animal fat from their product completely. Animal products were, after all, the competition. The problem was that cottonseed oil was liquid at room temperature, so making it behave like butter or cooking fat (lard) was impossible without mixing in some animal fat. And that remained a significant problem until 1911, when a little soap company called Procter & Gamble perfected a method of solidifying the cottonseed oil using hydrogen injection under pressure, or hydrogenation. Their fake shortening product, Crisco, a hydrogenated seed oil, took the market by storm. It was a fraction of the price of products based on animal fat but behaved pretty much the same way as lard when used as an ingredient.

The market for cheap seed-oil-based fat exploded. By 1967 seed-oil fats (which by then included soybean, corn, cottonseed, safflower and sunflower oils) accounted for 86 per cent of the fat consumed in the United States. Before Procter & Gamble's little foray out of soap and into food just six decades earlier, more than 90 per cent of the fat consumed by Americans had come from animals.

A big factor in the success of seed oils was their health halo. Right from the beginning Crisco had been marketed as a healthy alternative to animal fat. This was based on, well, nothing (those were the good old days in the advertising game). This message had stuck but after the Second World War it got an almighty boost from something that could have been a publicity disaster for the seed-oil industry. America was in the grip of a heart disease epidemic. In 1925, just 40 in every 100,000 men aged 55–64 died of heart disease. By 1950 that number was 600 in 100,000. A fifteenfold increase in just 25 years was catastrophic, but it became really important when President Eisenhower was struck down with a heart attack in 1955. He survived that first attack and was put on a highly publicised diet that included fake fats. Seed-oil-based health claims had just received presidential endorsement.

The perverse thing is that animal fats copped the blame for a disease that had only really become a significant problem during the three decades the United States had been steadily replacing animal fats with seed oils. By rights, seed-oil manufacturers should have been defending themselves rather than receiving the presidential tick of approval. Unfortunately (for us), the newly minted profession of human nutrition made its first big call and blamed a modern epidemic on an ancient food. Modern science now tells us that it was a catastrophically bad call (see below), but it didn't stop the seed-oil industry riding that pony for all it was worth.

The polyunsaturated-oil industry exploded. We'd been advised that animal fat was bad but vegetable fat was good, so we demanded that anyone selling us food make it 'healthy' by getting rid of the animal fat. And we didn't stop at margarine and cooking fat. By the late 1990s in the United States and the mid-2000s in Australia, we were even turning 'junk food' into 'health food'. First McDonald's, and then slowly everybody else, stopped using animal fat to fry food. The seed-oiling of our diet was complete. By the time you read these words you'll find it almost impossible to buy food containing animal fat from a supermarket, a restaurant or a takeaway joint. The only real exception is milk-based products, but even they are under threat because of what the cows are being fed (a story for later – read on, McDuff).

Unfortunately, as you're about to see, the consequences for us have been disastrous.

Omega-3 and omega-6 fats

Modern biochemistry tells us that saturated fats are critical to the proper operation of the machine we walk around in. It also tells us that if we mess with the mix of fats we consume, we can significantly affect important systems in our body. When we look closely at how our body processes and uses fats, the truth about dietary fats becomes abundantly clear. The advice we have been and continue to be given is not just wrong, it's seriously endangering our health.

Our bodies can make only two kinds of fat: saturated and monounsaturated. This is why 92 per cent of the fat in our bodies is one or the other of those two types. The other 8 per cent should be fats based on the polyunsaturated fats we get from our diet, the so-called 'essential fatty acids' (essential because we need them and we can't make them). The two main polyunsaturated fatty acids our bodies can't manufacture are linoleic acid (an omega-6 fat) and alpha-linolenic acid (ALA, an omega-3). You don't need to remember those names. From now on I'll just refer to them as omega-3 and omega-6.

We use omega-3 and omega-6 fats as critical components of our eyes, as messengers in our central nervous system, and to manufacture other types of polyunsaturated fats, the hormone-like molecules we use to control many of our systems (mainly inflammation and immunity). But we only need a maximum of 3 per cent (and perhaps as little as 1 per cent) of the calories we consume to be made up of these essential fatty acids. And, as for most things in our bodies, we need the balance to be just right. If we have just the right amount of both, then everything hums along. But if we push out the balance between them or have too many of them in total, we start to encounter the serious problems set out below.

It's difficult to know with certainty how much omega-3 and omega-6 we need, but scientists examining remaining hunter-gatherer populations peg the number at around 1.5 grams per day of each. Those populations manage to get that amount from their normal whole-food diet and don't suffer any diseases associated with deficiencies in those essential fats. It's reasonable, based on those population studies, to assume that once upon a time, most humans consumed about 3 grams of polyunsaturated fat a day (less than a teaspoonful) and that was about half omega-3 and half omega-6. We also know that once grains became a significant part of the human diet 10,000–12,000 years ago, the amount of omega-6 doubled to around 3 grams per day with no significant ill effects.

Before the invention of seed oils, we obtained omega-3 and omega-6 from our everyday diet without any great difficulty because just about every whole food contains some of each. Grains and nuts (and the flesh of some animals that eat them) are higher in omega-6 fats, while grasses and algae (and the flesh of animals and fish that eat them) are higher in omega-3 fats. And while you could easily get more than enough by subsisting on nuts (or lamb chops), there's really no need to seek out these fats specially. According to US Department of Agriculture statistics, we eat almost exactly the same amount of omega-3 fats today as we did in 1909. Here are a couple of lists of everyday foods and the amounts (in grams per 100 grams) of omega-3 and omega-6 fats they contain. Remember, we only need 1.5 grams of each.

Sources of omega-3 (arranged from highest Omega-3 to lowest)

Real food	Omega-3	Omega-6
Walnuts, raw	6.3	43.3
Mustard powder, dry	4.6	7.3
Mutton, casserole, separable fat, raw	2.0	2.2
Pacific king salmon fillets, flesh only, raw	1.8	0.2
Soybeans, dried	1.6	11.0
Mutton, all cuts, separable fat, cooked	1.0	1.6
Lamb, all cuts, separable fat, cooked	0.9	1.1
Lamb loin, separable fat, grilled	0.9	1.1
Rabbit flesh, casseroled	0.8	0.7
Haricot beans, dried	0.8	0.5
Beef dripping	0.8	2.0
Pork loin roast, separable fat, raw	0.7	9.4
Ghee (clarified butter)	0.7	1.3
Red kidney beans, dried	0.6	0.4
Pecans, unsalted	0.6	24.3
Lamb tongue, simmered	0.6	0.6
Lamb liver, grilled	0.6	0.7
Chicken, separable fat, composite, raw	0.6	7.4
Beef tail, simmered	0.5	0.4

This list and the one that follows were assembled from the free access database of more than 2000 foods that appears at davidgillespie.org/product_list. So if your favourite food isn't on the list, head over to the database and you'll probably find it and its exact content of omega-3 and omega-6 (and fructose, just for good measure). You'll see a few foods on both lists. The descending order is the important bit, not that there are foods in common. Looking at the table on page 52 of omega-6, you can see straight away that walnuts need to be eaten sparingly. Looking at the second table, you'll see that while walnuts are good for omega-3 they carry a motherload of omega-6.

Sources of omega-6 (arranged in order from highest omega-6 to lowest)

Real food	Omega-6	Omega-3
Walnuts, raw	43.3	6.3
Pine nuts, raw	39.8	—
Sunflower seeds	34.5	—
Brazil nuts, raw or blanched	29.0	—
Tahini (sesame seed pulp)	27.9	0.1
Sesame seeds, white	24.4	
Pecans, unsalted	24.3	0.6
Pumpkin seeds, hulled and dried	20.6	0.2
Pistachio nuts, unsalted	15.8	—
Peanuts, with skin, raw	15.0	—
Almonds, with skin	12.8	—
Soybeans, dried	11.0	1.6
Palm oil	9.1	0.2
Olive oil	8.3	0.5
Pork loin roast, separable fat, roasted	8.2	0.6
Cashew nuts, raw	7.5	—
Mustard powder, dry	7.3	4.6
Hazelnuts, raw	7.0	0.1
Duck, skin and fat, raw	6.5	0.4
Pork loin chop, separable fat, dry-fried	5.9	0.4
Margarine, cooking	5.7	0.7
Pork forequarter, separable fat, barbecued	5.6	0.5
Chicken, separable fat from multiple parts of the chicken, baked	5.5	0.2
Duck, skin and fat, baked	5.3	0.3
Bacon, middle rasher, untrimmed grilled	5.2	0.4

Omega-6 fats are the primary ingredients of seed oils, which means that now seed oils are used in just about every commercially produced food, the amount of omega-6 oils we consume has exploded. We would obtain almost twice our daily requirement of omega-6 fat from just one small serve of KFC chips (2.74 grams); and a third of our daily requirement of omega-3 fat (0.54 grams) from the same serve. While most of us are probably getting just enough omega-3, we're all getting vast amounts of omega-6 if we eat polyunsaturated seed oils or anything made with them – which is an awful lot of things.

HOW MUCH POLYUNSATURATED FAT SHOULD WE EAT?

It's hard to put an exact figure on it, but it's likely we require around 1.5 grams of omega-3 and 1.5 grams of omega-6 every day. In today's food environment you'll easily hit that number for each type of fat. You won't need to supplement with omega-3 if you Eat Real Food. And as long as you're judicious with your use of nuts and seeds, you won't go too far north of 1.5 grams of omega-6. Even if you do overshoot, there's no evidence to suggest you'll be doing harm at even twice that number. So, the rule of thumb I use is that we should aim for our polyunsaturated-fat consumption to be between 3 and 6 grams per day.

The seven ways polyunsaturated fats will hurt you

In the pages that follow I give a quick tour of what we know about the harm caused by large amounts of these polyunsaturated fats, but if you don't want to know the details, here's the list.

The seven ways polyunsaturated fat will hurt you

1. Polyunsaturated fats cause cancer.
2. Polyunsaturated fats help fructose cause heart disease.
3. Polyunsaturated fats make you blind.
4. Polyunsaturated fats cause Parkinson's disease.
5. Polyunsaturated fats give you rheumatoid arthritis and other autoimmune diseases.
6. Polyunsaturated fats give you osteoporosis.
7. Polyunsaturated fats cause allergies and asthma.

Once again, there are two main disease clusters initiated by too much polyunsaturated fat. Those fats are easily oxidised, so when they're incorporated into our cell membranes or transported in our bloodstream, they eventually result in cancer, macular degeneration and heart disease. The other disease group relates to omega-6 in particular. These fats are used by our immune system to promote inflammation and other immune responses. It's early days in the research on this, but it's increasingly likely that they're responsible for diseases as diverse as Parkinson's disease and rheumatoid arthritis, and may even play a significant role in other autoimmune diseases, such as multiple sclerosis and lupus. But let's start with the one disease that affects almost all of us directly or indirectly, and the one for which we have explicit high-quality evidence of harm from human trials. Cancer.

1 Polyunsaturated fats cause cancer

Between 1985 and 2000, the rate of new prostate cancers in Australia increased by 15 per cent a year. Breast cancer increased

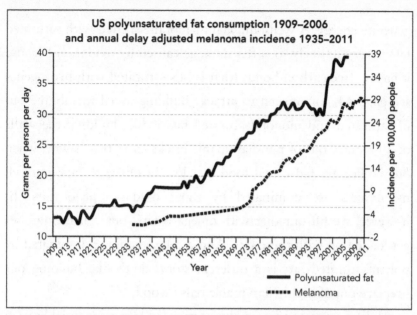

US polyunsaturated fat consumption 1909–2006 and annual delay adjusted melanoma incidence 1935–2011

In Australia the equivalent rates are significantly higher. In 2000, the incidence of melanoma among Australian men (53.7 per 100,000) was more than twice the US rate. The incidence of melanoma has accelerated in lock step with polyunsaturated-fat consumption for the last 70 years. Is it really sensible to suggest the average American is getting 25 times as much sun now as they were in 1933?

by 37 per cent. And melanoma increased by 60 per cent in men and 22 per cent in women. During that period we all ate less saturated fat and more polyunsaturated fat than ever before in the long history of our species on this planet.

We've grown up thinking of oxygen as our friend. When someone is injured they're often given oxygen. And it's what's in the tanks feeding those masks we hope will never drop from an aircraft ceiling. But to most cells in our body, oxygen is both life-giving and a very dangerous substance. And this is because oxygen is highly reactive. Every cell in our body has a membrane made of fat. Inside each of those cells we use oxygen's reactivity to 'burn' glucose and generate energy. A well-built cell membrane stuffed with saturated fats is very unlikely to suffer damage caused by oxidation because it has no free carbon bonds (that is, it's saturated with hydrogen – see page 44) for oxygen to attack. Building a cell membrane out of saturated and monounsaturated fats is like building the walls of a fireplace out of non-flammable bricks. And this is why, when our bodies are fed a real food diet low in omega-6 fats, our cell membranes are dominated by those oxidation-proof fats. If, however, we fill our diet with omega-6 fats, our cell membranes get loaded up with these fats. And a cell membrane dominated by polyunsaturated fats is a different story: that's like building our fireplace out of highly flammable balsa wood.

Unlike saturated fats, polyunsaturated fats react quickly with oxygen. This is a very, very bad thing in a body that needs to be as oxygen-resistant as possible. And when oxygen reacts with polyunsaturated fat, it breaks that fat down into a range of dangerous chemicals. In the process, it destroys the integrity of any cell made from fat – which is every cell in our body. If you eat a real food diet then this really won't be a problem. Yes, some of the omega-6 you eat will end up oxidised in your cell membranes, but it won't be much and what little there is will be efficiently dealt with by your body's homegrown antioxidants (our own little fire brigade).

But when we eat a lot of omega-6 fat it causes massive ongoing oxidation. This overwhelms our antioxidant fire brigade, which leads to significant damage to the cell membrane and can damage a cell all the way down to the DNA.

Our cells normally die and replicate according to a schedule. They have DNA switches that tell them when they should replicate and when to die. If those DNA switches are damaged by oxidation on a massive scale, then the damaged cells can become a breeding ground for potential cancer growth.

We can compensate for DNA damage and most of it does no permanent harm at all. But every now and then, DNA damage produces a mutation that would help the next generation of cells become cancerous. Cancerous cells don't respond to the normal genetic signals telling them to stop replicating, and their programmed cell death doesn't function as it should. They can persuade the surrounding tissue to provide them with a blood supply, they can trick our immune system into not seeing them as a threat (they are, after all, our own cells), and worst of all they can invade our blood or lymphatic system and travel to other places in the body (this is called metastasis and it makes most cancers almost impossible to treat).

Obviously, the more times a cell replicates the greater the chance of the 'right' mutation arising. This has recently been confirmed in research that demonstrates (mathematically) that the biggest determinant of the likelihood of a cancer in any part of the body is the number of times the cells in that organ normally replicate. So our lifetime risk of bowel cancer and melanoma is high because those cells replicate the most frequently. And our lifetime risk of cancers in our limbs or gall bladder are low because those cells replicate the least often.

The same study also demonstrated that we can significantly increase that lifetime risk. The researchers had good data on smoking and were able to show that even though (of course) cells in the lung replicate at the same rate in smokers and non-smokers, the lifetime risk of cancer in smokers was much higher.

The smokers had introduced a substance that caused more DNA damage in lung cells and the result was a massive increase in cancer risk.

It takes billions of random, chaotic collapses of oxidised cells to produce cells with the ability to form tumours. Our bodies need to be exposed to oxidation over very long time frames, but if they are, they could eventually produce the mutations that are lumped together under the general heading 'cancer'. If we introduce a substance into the cell membrane (such as omega-6) that significantly increases the chances of cell death and DNA damage through oxidation, then we are, just as the smoker did, massively increasing the likelihood that cancers will form. The difference is that this risk increase applies to all cells (not just the lung cells) because it affects every cell in our body.

This is not just a pretty hypothesis. We know for certain that, in rats, dietary omega-6 fats rapidly accelerate the growth and spread of breast cancers. In humans, study after study is coming to the same conclusion. Higher omega-6 fat consumption usually doubles the risk of breast cancer. That's true in the United States (80 per cent increased risk), Sweden (83 per cent), Mexico (92 per cent), Israel (100 per cent), China (106 per cent), France (131 per cent), and Singapore (145 per cent).

And it's not just breast cancer. A randomised controlled trial in US men reported a near doubling in deaths from all cancers in the group whose diet was 15 per cent omega-6 fats when compared to a control group for whom it was 5 per cent. And a similar study in France showed that when the trial group reduced their omega-6 fats (from 5.3 per cent of calories to 3.6 per cent), cancer rates were also reduced (by 61 per cent).

The risk of cancer has always been with us and always will be with us. It's a consequence of having cells that replicate imperfectly. But omega-6 consumption at least doubles (and probably significantly increases even more) our chances of becoming a victim. When we layer in some of the other disease trajectories I've been discussing, we change cancer from a possibility to a probability. One in three Australians over the age of 50 now takes statins (drugs to lower their blood cholesterol, an important suppressor of cell damage through oxidation – see *Big Fat Lies* for a lengthy discussion). But a side effect of taking them is that they also shut down our production of coenzyme Q10, one of the important antioxidants produced by our liver (see the next section for more detail). So not only are we consuming a substance that significantly increases our need for antioxidants, but many of us are also simultaneously taking a drug that destroys our ability to produce them. Worse than that, recent research suggests that omega-6 also directly disables one of our genetic defences against cancer (the BRCA gene). Add to that fructose's ability to provide the DNA elements necessary for tumour growth, and you have the perfect recipe for cancer.

Current health advice targets cholesterol and saturated fat. We're told to eat margarine instead of butter, eat low-fat foods (which replace the fat with sugar) and take cholesterol-lowering drugs. The combined consequence of this advice is a massive increase in oxidative damage, removal of our defences to that damage (in multiple ways) and the creation of the building blocks for tumour growth. The current health advice is a perfect blueprint for cancer, and we've followed this blueprint to the letter.

With a food supply stuffed to the brim with both fructose and omega-6 fat, it's little wonder that our lifetime risk of contracting cancer now sits at one in two for men and one in three for women.

2 Polyunsaturated fats help fructose cause heart disease

Seed oils and sugar might be a terrific way to increase our odds of developing cancer, but there's an even more deadly disease that little combo brings to the table. The research now clearly shows that the oxidation of small dense LDL particles (rather than the mere consumption of dietary cholesterol) is the primary cause of heart disease. The very best way to have that sort of particle in your bloodstream is to eat sugar and the very best way to ensure it's oxidised is to eat omega-6 fats.

As we saw in Chapter 2, people can be divided into two main groups according to whether their LDL particles are mostly large and fluffy or smaller and less fluffy. The folks with the large, fluffy particles are said to be pattern A and those with smaller, less fluffy particles are pattern B. We know that the best way to convert someone from pattern A to pattern B is to feed them lots of fructose.

Which LDL pattern you are matters, because if you're pattern A, your LDL reading is not an indicator of heart disease risk. But pattern B people have a heart disease risk three times that of pattern A people. This is because pattern A LDL particles are much less prone to oxidation. The more cholesterol an LDL particle has, the larger and more buoyant (fluffy) it is and the less likely it is to oxidise. Pattern B LDL particles are deficient in cholesterol and therefore much more prone to oxidation.

It might be helpful to think of LDL particles as trucks used to transport fat from the liver to the cells that need them. They need to transport their cargo through a bloodstream full of oxygen. If their cargo is saturated fat then that's not too much of a problem, because it won't react with the oxygen. But if it's a polyunsaturated fat then it will. Not to worry, though, our cargo trucks can cope with a little bit of oxygen en route because they're also loaded up with antioxidants (think of them as fire extinguishers on trucks with a flammable cargo) for the trip. These antioxidants include vitamin E, coenzyme Q10 and cholesterol (which also inhibits oxidation). Unfortunately, if we consume large quantities of polyunsaturated fats and transport them in substandard trucks (pattern B) we'll quickly overwhelm our in-built safeguards against oxidation.

An oxidised LDL particle is like a truck with its load on fire. It's careering down our bloodstream highway with burnt bits and pieces of polyunsaturated fat. Some of them become embedded in our arterial walls, because nitric oxide (which is meant to stop that happening) has been depleted by fructose (see Chapter 2). Our immune system regards these damaged trucks as a danger to the body and immediately swings into action to dispose of them. As our little defenders (the macrophages of our innate immune system) ingest these damaged particles, they themselves become part of the problem, clumping together, full of fat cells and other debris, in the arterial wall. Those clumps eventually form the plaques that are the hallmark of heart disease. If you've seen a highway blocked by emergency service vehicles attending an accident, you know exactly how our bloodstream looks when our immune system attends the scene of an oxidised LDL incident.

Once again the unforeseen consequences of the advice to decrease saturated fat and not worry about sugar have meant that the disease that advice explicitly targets (heart disease) has been made much worse rather than better.

3 Polyunsaturated fats make you blind

Macular degeneration is the primary cause of blindness in Australia today. One in seven Australians over the age of 50 (a little over a million people) has the disease, and this number is likely to increase by at least 70 per cent by 2030.

The macula, at the centre of our retina, contains the very specialised rod and cone cells that allow us to see in fine detail and in colour respectively. These cells are unusual in that they use polyunsaturated fats in their membranes rather than the saturated and monounsaturated fats used by most of our other cells. If our macula is damaged, we can no longer see fine detail, meaning we're likely to have trouble reading, driving, recognising faces and so on. The rod and cone cells use omega-3 polyunsaturated fats precisely because they oxidise when exposed to light. The oxidation of these fats is an important part of how our eyes work. Naturally, this means that our eyes are spectacularly well adapted to dealing with the oxidised rubbish created when we 'burn' omega-3 polyunsaturated fats. Our eyes contain a specialised immune system that reacts to some of the more dangerous waste products produced by the process. Unfortunately, though, it seems our eyes are not too choosy about which polyunsaturated fats they use. If our diet is high in omega-6 fats then those get used instead of the omega-3s. And that wouldn't matter much except that the junk-clearing immune system doesn't seem to recognise junk produced from omega-6 fats.

When the eye's waste disposal system fails, we accumulate junk deposits in our eyes called drusen. Drusen are visible in an eye examination and are a sure sign of the development of macular degeneration. It's highly likely that the blame for the massive increases in the number of Australians with the disease can be laid squarely at the feet of the companies filling our food with omega-6 fat. If you'd like more detail on the exact processes involved and the current research on macular degeneration, then please take a look at my book *Toxic Oil*.

Consumption of omega-6 fat for its supposed heart-health benefits is not only harming our heart and causing cancer, but also driving the epidemic of macular degeneration that now engulfs Australia.

4 Polyunsaturated fats cause Parkinson's disease

James Parkinson, surgeon, geologist and palaeontologist, first described what we now call Parkinson's disease in his paper on shaking palsy in 1817. Dr Parkinson described a condition that causes involuntary tremors when a limb is at rest, rigidity, slowness of movement, and a propensity to bend forwards and a slow gait when walking. We now know that Parkinson's is caused by the death of cells in our pars compacta – the part of our brain that controls motor function (the substantia nigra pars compacta, if you want to get all technical). That part of the brain is a central switching room for movement, attention, learning and reward-seeking (which makes sure we keep eating and having sex).

The pars compacta exerts its control using a hormone called dopamine. When everything is working well, our body is inhibited from moving by the part of our brain that contains the pars compacta (the basal ganglia for Latin freaks). When we decide to move something (our eyes or limbs, and so on), the pars compacta squirts out dopamine to take the brakes off. If the neurons responsible for producing the dopamine are damaged, not enough dopamine is produced and the brakes don't come off. Parkinson's disease is the result. Our brain is pretty durable, because we lose around 50 per cent of our dopamine-manufacturing neurons before showing any symptoms. But once they're gone, these neurons are gone forever. As the numbers of neurons decrease, a Parkinson's sufferer has to exert greater and greater conscious effort to produce movement.

The only effective treatment for Parkinson's is medication that can increase dopamine production by squeezing a little more out of the remaining neurons. Obviously, if the destruction of the neurons continues (as it does in most people) that's only a temporary solution. Before medication was introduced in the 1970s, a Parkinson's patient was expected to live nine and a half years after diagnosis. The drug-assisted life expectancy is now fifteen years.

Because the disease is the result of cumulative destruction, it's most prevalent in people over 50, but 20 per cent of cases are diagnosed between twenty and 50. Michael J. Fox was diagnosed when he was just 30. There are very few places in the world where accurate long-term statistics have been kept on the incidence of Parkinson's disease, but they have done just that in Olmsted County, Minnesota (population 147,066). There, researchers have concluded, annual new cases almost doubled between 1944 and 1984 (using consistent diagnostic rules). And, as for type 2 diabetes, other studies tell us that Parkinson's occurs much less frequently among populations not exposed to a Western diet (processed food).

We know that a diet high in seed oils causes the levels of omega-6 fats in our cell membranes to rise rapidly. Those fats react quickly with oxygen and push the body into a state of cascading cell damage called oxidative stress. We also know that a major product of the oxidation of omega-6 fats is something with the charming name 4-hydroxynonenal (I'll just use its street name, 4-HNE). And we know that 4-HNE, while generally dangerous, is especially toxic to the neurons responsible for producing dopamine in our brain. Eating seed oils (or anything that contains large amounts of omega-6 fats) induces production of the 4-HNE molecule that kills the neurons we depend upon for dopamine production. Kill enough of them and you have Parkinson's disease.

5 Polyunsaturated fats give you rheumatoid arthritis and other autoimmune diseases

Every day, seventeen Australians have a joint replaced because of rheumatoid arthritis (RA). And the number of us with the disease is accelerating quickly, particularly among children. There are more than 100 types of arthritis, but RA is the most severe and the second most common (after osteoarthritis). Unlike osteoarthritis, RA is not caused by wear and tear on the joints (often from being overweight, exercising too much or both). Rather, it's an autoimmune disease, like type 1 diabetes, multiple sclerosis, lupus and asthma.

An RA sufferer's immune-system inflammation response is malfunctioning, causing it to attack the synovial membrane, the tissues lining our joints. The synovial membrane is normally very thin. Its job is to produce fluid that lubricates and nourishes the joint. The immune-system attack causes the synovial membrane to become swollen and inflamed. Over time this leads to bone damage in the joint and eventually irreversible joint damage.

Australia doesn't keep good data on any chronic disease, but as of 2007, there were approximately 428,000 sufferers of RA, about two-thirds of whom were women. It can affect anyone and is most prevalent in people over 40, but it's increasingly affecting children. About a quarter of RA sufferers experience severe pain on a daily basis and more than half of sufferers need to stop work within ten years of onset of the disease. Hospitalisation for RA (largely for joint replacement) has been steadily increasing. The rate doubled in the first decade of the 21st century. Alarmingly, it appears that the incidence is increasing even more rapidly in children, for whom the rate of hospitalisation more than tripled over the same time frame.

Researchers have known for some time that the omega-6 and omega-3 polyunsaturated fats are critical to the way our inflammation response works, particularly when it comes to RA. Omega-6 fats dial it up and omega-3 fats dial it back down again.

Analysis of the inflamed synovial membrane in RA patients reveals that it's very high in molecules derived from omega-6 fats. Knowing that omega-3 and omega-6 fats act on inflammation in opposite ways, researchers have conducted trials in rats. These show that artificially induced RA can be significantly delayed or eliminated if the rats are fed fish oil (high in omega-3 fats) rather than vegetable oil (high in omega-6 fats). That research has led to large numbers of controlled human trials that have successfully reduced RA inflammation (and associated pain) by supplementing with omega-3 fats (usually from fish oil).

Given those results, it would be almost impossible to get ethical approval for a trial that tried to make RA worse by feeding people omega-6, but one trial figured out a different way to skin the cat. In that trial researchers increased the amount of omega-3 they fed the subjects while also dividing them into groups, one a standard Western diet and one on a diet very low in omega-6 fats. The results of the trial were impressively in favour of the RA patients on the low-omega-6 diet (and even better if they also took fish oil).

The science is old and uncontroversial. The massive increase in omega-6 fats in the Western diet makes us much more likely to suffer from RA and will make RA worse once we have it. The problem is that in Australia today it's almost impossible to buy packaged food that isn't infused with these RA-inducing fats.

As debilitating as RA is, it's just one of a series of diseases on the same autoimmunity spectrum. Like RA, multiple sclerosis (MS) is caused by our immune system attacking part of our body, namely myelin, the fatty sheath that serves as the electrical insulation for our brain, spinal cord and nerves. Or, to be more specific, it is the cells that produce our myelin that are destroyed by our immune system. Over time, the accumulated damage results in our neurons losing function and being no longer able to communicate. This results in an array of symptoms as diverse as lowered cognitive function, depression, tremors, blindness and bowel dysfunction, to name just a few.

We know that the proximate cause of the autoimmune attack is a failure of that part of our immune system responsible for shutting down our immune response – known as the T-regulatory cells (or just T-regs). We also know that two things in particular will degrade T-reg function: omega-6 fat consumption and a fatty liver. So a really excellent way to get an out-of-control immune response underway is to eat loads of omega-6 fats and sugar (which as we saw in Chapter 2 causes fatty liver) – in other words, eat fake food.

But there's an even more insidious connection to MS than an overactive immune response. One of the oddest things statisticians have observed about MS is that if you move from a country with a low rate of MS to one with a high MS rate after you turn twenty, your likelihood of contracting MS doesn't increase. But if you do it when you're younger, you acquire the risk level of the country you move to.

The process of coating our brain and spinal cord in myelin is incomplete when we're born. In fact, it's barely started. It takes us about 25 years to get the job fully done. We know that omega-6 fats deactivate the cells that produce the myelin. If during those first 25 years we're exposed to significant quantities of omega-6 fats, we may be laying the groundwork for immune-system attacks later in life. That's speculation at the moment, but when it comes to my kids, I don't take the risk.

Similar mechanisms appear to be at play in many autoimmune diseases, all of which lead to horrible lifelong degradations of life quality. The likely involvement of omega-6 fats in these diseases provides reason enough (if more were needed) to avoid such fats.

6 Polyunsaturated fats give you osteoporosis

Scientists have known for more than a decade that the omega-6 fats in vegetable oils degrade human bone density. Now new research has thrown light on how that happens and why anyone concerned about osteoporosis needs to stop consuming these fats immediately.

One in twenty Australians has osteoporosis (Greek for 'porous bones'), one in four has low bone density (the precursor to osteoporosis) and the number of people affected is accelerating wildly. In the last ten years the number of GP visits in Australia related to osteoporosis has doubled.

Our bones are not static lumps of rock. They are living tissue that constantly accumulate and dispose of minerals. Osteoporosis occurs when bones lose minerals, such as calcium, more quickly than the body can replace them, causing a loss of bone thickness (bone density or mass).

As bones become thinner and less dense, even a minor bump or fall can cause a serious fracture. Unfortunately, most people don't know they have the disease until they suffer a break. Eight out of ten cases are recorded in people over the age of 55, but the age of onset is becoming progressively younger.

Osteoporosis medicines work by making the cells that break down bone (osteoclasts) less active. This tips the balance towards accumulation of minerals by the cells that form bone (osteoblasts).

A long series of animal studies has clearly established that polyunsaturated fats are important drivers of the bone-recycling process. We know that the polyunsaturated omega-3s that predominate in some fish oils, flaxseeds and kelp help us build up bone density, while the omega-6 oils that predominate in seed oils (such as sunflower, soybean, canola, safflower and rice bran oil) destroy bone density.

In 2005 researchers at the University of California confirmed that the same rules were at work in a large human population.

In that study, 1532 people were observed for four years. The results were spectacularly consistent. The more omega-6 a person consumed (or the higher their omega-6 to omega-3 ratio), the lower their bone density. It really was that black and white. The results were independent of medication use, so even the drugs didn't save the participants from the effects of the omega-6 fats.

Unfortunately (for our health), nobody in the health community wants to hear that they should stop telling people to eat vegetable oils, so there's been precious little publicity about that line of studies. That is, until bone density started mattering to people who breed animals for a living.

As we feed more and more of our farmed fish diets that are high in omega-6 fats, they're becoming more and more fragile. It seems that just like humans (and rats), their bones go to pot if we ramp up the omega-6. This latest proof of the bone-destroying power of omega-6 comes courtesy of a 2014 aquaculture study by the Norwegian National Institute of Nutrition and Seafood Research. The scientists observed a rise in the level of activity of the enzyme that breaks down bone, in line with the rise in omega-6 concentrations.

We don't know exactly how omega-6 works its destructive magic, but the research so far suggests it might lie on a completely different disease spectrum from either the oxidation effect, which leads to heart disease and cancer, or the inflammation effect, which leads to autoimmune diseases. Scientists suspect it relates to the production of PGE_2, the prostaglandin responsible for bone metabolism. We make PGE_2 from omega-6 fats, but the presence of omega-3 fats stops it being produced. If we make just the right amount everything is tickety-boo, but if we make too much because, say, we have too much omega-6 and not enough omega-3, then we start breaking down our bones. We also know that PGE$_2$ production is affected by the presence or absence of oestrogen, and that might go some considerable way to explaining why osteoporosis disproportionately affects women.

7 Polyunsaturated fats cause allergies and asthma

For more, see 'Polyunsaturated fats cause allergies and asthma in children' below.

The four ways sugar and polyunsaturated fats can harm an unborn child

I started looking at sugar because I'm a self-obsessed male – so pretty average, really – who wanted to be thinner. Once I broke my addiction to sugar I could calmly assess the rest of what I was shoving in my gob. Addicts just want to eat anything, but we real-food eaters are a lot more discerning and (because we're not addicted to food) can choose to go without if necessary. That dispassionate look at the research led me to discover the dangers of industrial fats and made me want very much to steer clear of them, too. But as I read deeper into the research, I discovered more and more aspects of eating sugar and fats that should concern any parent or prospective parent. A great deal of the damage done by these substances is intergenerational. What a mother eats during pregnancy and while breastfeeding can profoundly influence the life and health of her child. This section provides an overview of the four ways that sugar and polyunsaturated fat will harm your unborn child. Obviously, for the purposes of this list, I'm assuming that women have not consumed so much fructose as to render them infertile and men have not consumed enough to destroy their erectile function.

1 Fructose sets your children up for obesity

During the last decade, researchers have become increasingly interested in the intergenerational transmission of obesity and type 2 diabetes. Rat studies have repeatedly confirmed that feeding offspring fructose while they're suckling (the rat equivalent of breastfeeding) – even after they're weaned – will make them more susceptible to obesity and type 2 diabetes if they're later exposed to fructose. But an even more recent study has demonstrated that the damage begins with what the mother is eating. In that study, one group of lactating female rats was given access to water that was 10 per cent sugar (the same as a soft drink) and compared to controls that just drank water. Both groups ate the same rat chow. A bunch of tests were then run on them and their offspring. The mother rats that drank sugar while lactating didn't put on any more weight than those drinking water. But it was a different story altogether for their offspring. Disturbingly, their endocrine (hormone) systems showed deep dysfunction. After weaning, they weighed more and ate more than the offspring of the control rats, even though they'd never been exposed to fructose. Worse, they were significantly more likely to gain weight into adulthood and significantly more likely to suffer insulin resistance (the precursor to type 2 diabetes). These studies haven't been tried in humans, but the researchers were confident that – as for other rat studies involving fructose that have been replicated in people – the results are likely to apply to us. If that's so, it means that a breastfeeding mother who consumes fructose is likely condemning her children to (at least) obesity and type 2 diabetes, even if those children never touch a gram of sugar.

BREASTFEEDING IS BEST

You could come away from reading these sections and conclude that breastfeeding is dangerous but that is emphatically not the case. What these studies show is that what a mother eats while she breastfeeds is critically important. Human breastmilk is an extraordinarily complex food that delivers exactly the right nutrients at exactly the time a baby needs them. In comparison, formula is a very blunt and poorly designed instrument. If you can breastfeed, it's always the best option, but be very careful of your diet while you do it.

---

2 Polyunsaturated-fat consumption by breastfeeding mothers increases the risk of breast cancer in their daughters

We know that the omega-6 fats in vegetable oils increase the risk of breast cancer in the person consuming the oil, but some studies are starting to show that this risk is also transmitted to that person's daughters. Rat studies performed in the 1970s and 1980s consistently noted that mammary (breast) cancer occurred more often among rats fed corn oil (which is high in polyunsaturated fats) than among those fed coconut oil (which is high in saturated fats). But a truly disturbing study published in 1997 showed that feeding the suckling mother rat a diet high in polyunsaturated fat (43 per cent corn oil) doubled the rate of mammary cancer in her daughters, caused cancers to appear among them earlier and caused earlier onset of puberty. There are no human studies to back that up (I think you'd struggle with ethical approval where your hypothesis is that feeding people margarine gives them breast cancer). But at the population level, we know that Australian women are eating more vegetable oil and getting more breast cancer at a younger age, and that the average age for the onset of puberty is decreasing.

3 Polyunsaturated fats are critical to the growth of our brain and nervous system

A significant component of what makes us intelligent is created from our mother's fat stores. Unfortunately, the omega-6 fats that predominate in margarines and processed food stop that absorption happening and impair intelligence in children. If you want your kids to be as smart as they can be, then they (and you) need to stop eating those fats immediately.

About 10 per cent of our brain is made from an omega-3 fat called DHA (docosahexaenoic acid for the biochemists among us). We can make DHA from a simpler omega-3 fat called ALA (alpha-linolenic acid). That's the form of omega-3 that exists in most of our food. Unfortunately, less than 0.5 per cent of the ALA we consume ends up as DHA. This means that relying on mum to eat enough omega-3 ALA while she's pregnant would be a disastrous strategy for building a baby's brain. Luckily, our bodies have a plan. As soon as a woman reaches puberty her body starts storing up as much omega-3 fat as it can. Uniquely among animals (because we're the only ones who need to build relatively gigantic brains), female humans store all that omega-3 ALA in a baby pantry located at the top of the legs and in the buttocks.

Unfortunately for girls who wish to become supermodels, the body can't tell the difference between the various sorts of fat, so it just stores all the fat it can find in the hope that enough of it will be the good stuff. Since the point of storing the fat is to ensure there's enough ALA to make DHA to make a baby's brain, the body won't let go of it easily. That is, until the third trimester of pregnancy. Then the floodgates are opened and the fat is released. Because brain construction doesn't finish when a child is born, it's also important that the supply of DHA continues after the baby is born. Breastmilk (and now formula) contains large amounts of DHA. In total, 80 per cent of the fat used in the construction of a child's brain comes from the mother's stores (rather than her current diet). So perhaps the old saying should be 'A moment on the lips, a lifetime in your child's brain'.

We know from animal studies that if there's not enough DHA, animals end up with brains that don't have enough neurons, the cells that do all the work in our brains. That lack of basic circuitry in turn impairs the offspring's development and intelligence. And it looks like the results hold in humans as well. Very recently, a study in humans showed that the amount of DHA in breastmilk was the strongest predictor of test performance across samples drawn from 28 OECD countries.

But before you start force-feeding teenage girls, mothers and kids fish oil tablets, you should know that there's a little twist in this tale. Omega-6 fats stop us using DHA to make us brainy. So it doesn't matter how much omega-3 you have if you also consume too much omega-6. Omega-6 fats compete with omega-3 fats for the same enzymes. Critically, one of those is the enzyme that turns garden-variety omega-3 ALA into DHA. If we have equal amounts of omega-3 and omega-6 in our diet, just the right amount of DHA is created and all is good, but if we have too much omega-6, we fail to make enough DHA.

You might predict from this that countries where people eat a lot of seed oils loaded with omega-6 would tend not to do so well in tests – and you'd be right. The most recent study found that there was a very strong correlation between the amount of omega-6 in the diet and how poorly fifteen-year-olds did on standard international benchmark tests. This confirmed the findings of five previous human studies, which showed that higher omega-6 intakes impaired cognition (made us dumb – translation provided in case you've been hitting the margarine). Indeed, one 2011 study determined that the impairment was greater than the effect of lead!! (Double exclamation marks are well and truly warranted on that statement.)

Just like omega-3 fats, omega-6 fats are stored in the baby pantry, ready to use when needed. So the fats used to construct a baby's brain are not just the fats a woman is eating when she's pregnant or breastfeeding. They're every fat she's stored since puberty (or since the last baby used them up). Babies being constructed today are having their brains built from the fats used in processed food for the last twenty years. We now use unleaded petrol because of the damage lead in petrol did to developing brains. If we want the next generation not to be 'cognitively impaired' by seed oils, we need to ensure that (at the very least) young women aren't consuming foods overloaded with omega-6 fats. In other words, they need to Eat Real Food. If they do this, their children will be smart enough to thank them for it.

4 Polyunsaturated fats cause allergies and asthma in children

One in four Australians now suffers from an allergic or immune disease, and the numbers are increasing at obscene rates. Reported rates of hay fever, asthma and eczema have doubled in the last fifteen years. Hospitalisation rates for the most extreme form of allergic reaction, anaphylaxis (life-threatening acute inflammation, usually in response to food), also doubled between 1994 and 2005. And the biggest overall change has been a fivefold increase in hospital admissions for children up to the age of four (as compared to just double for the rest of the population). That's a fivefold increase in just ten years! It's not your imagination, there's a lot more allergic disease around today than when you were a kid.

What all these diseases have in common is that they're part of our immune system's inflammatory response. Any injury or infection causes automatic and immediate inflammation. The swelling, pain, redness and heat are all functions of our inflammatory response. Without inflammation, wounds and infections would never heal. Our inflammation response is almost entirely controlled by substances derived from polyunsaturated fats. So when asthma and allergy rates started exploding, the logical place to look for an explanation was the massive increase in polyunsaturated fats in the diet.

Controlling that inflammation response is a very fine balancing act that depends on us having exactly the right amount and ratios of polyunsaturated fats in our diet. Small amounts of these oils are a critical component of our immune system, but overloading with them can push this system way out of balance. Chronic (or uncontrolled) inflammation leads to a host of diseases, including allergies and asthma.

An easily identifiable source of pro-inflammatory omega-6 fats in the diet is margarine. Scientists have conducted a number of large-scale trials to see if there's any relationship between margarine consumption and allergic disease. And guess what, trial after trial has concluded that children who consume more margarine have double the rate of medically diagnosed eczema, hay fever, allergies and asthma. This is true in Finnish children, and in German two-year-olds and three-year-olds 'liberated' by the fall of the Berlin Wall (and having the bad fortune to then be exposed to a diet containing margarine), among others.

Even when the kids themselves aren't chomping on margarine or vegetable oils, if their mother did during the last four weeks of pregnancy, they have at least a 50 per cent greater chance of having eczema, hay fever or allergies for life. To get to the bottom of why that might be, scientists have recently been comparing the amounts of polyunsaturated fats in a pregnant mother's umbilical cord blood supply (the unborn baby's food) to the likelihood of the child going on to develop chronic allergic disease. They've found a very direct relationship between the level of polyunsaturated fat in that blood supply and the risk of allergy. Not only that, the relationship is clearly dose-dependent. Want to give someone allergies, eczema, hay fever or asthma for life? Just increase the level of polyunsaturated fats. Want to decrease the risk? Just decrease the level of polyunsaturated fats. Simple.

Chronic allergies aren't a case of the sniffles and a mild rash. They can be (and increasingly are) lifelong sources of extreme and deadly danger. We now live in a society where a growing array of foods can kill us on contact and where asthma can snuff out a life just as efficiently. It's very rare that science (particularly nutrition science) provides an answer this unequivocal. Seed-oil consumption before or after birth causes lifelong allergic disease and asthma.

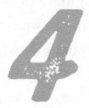

GRAINS AND SUPERFOODS: THE GOOD AND BAD NEWS

Grains or, more accurately, grass seeds, are a relatively new addition to the human diet. Not new in the same sense as sugar or seed oils, but new-ish. The human body you're walking around in was largely designed by the hunter-gatherer lifestyle we all enjoyed between 250,000 and 12,000 years ago and that some tribes still enjoy today. That period is the tail end of the Palaeolithic era (2.6 million years ago to 10,000 years ago). At that time, humans hadn't yet invented agriculture and, as a result, there were very few of us (around three million on the whole planet). Then we got the hang of making plants and animals give us food instead of us having to find it. That allowed us to change to the settled agricultural lifestyle almost every human on the planet enjoys today. Growing rather than finding food allowed us to increase our population significantly (there are now more than seven billion of us – 2333 times as many as when agriculture was invented) and gave us enormous advances in technology and culture more generally. You have more time to invent and enjoy stuff if you don't spend every hour of every day looking for something to eat.

While there have been definite advantages to the settled farming lifestyle, many people say that the change in diet it brought about is a high price to pay. Palaeolithic humans ate what was available. If they lived in a place with plentiful wild animals or fish they ate them (if they could catch and kill them with the simple weapons they had available) and supplemented their diet with any edible plants they could find. If they lived in a place with no animals they just ate the plants. We followed a simple rule. If something looked edible and didn't kill us instantly, it was food. And even though some modern aficionados of the 'Paleo' lifestyle like to emphasise the hunting part of the lifestyle (and assume that means they should eat loads of bacon and date-filled muffins, for some reason), in reality it was more like a gatherer-hunter way of life. Most of the food came from plants and it was supplemented with whatever animal or insect they could get hold of.

By the way, the human quirk of dividing the roles of hunting and gathering along gender lines is probably what allowed us to survive and prosper. Neanderthals (another human species) didn't do this and, as a result, lost a lot of women to the hunt (I'm reliably informed that bringing down a wild animal with a spear is extremely dangerous work) before they could produce children, meaning their population growth tended to be flat to negative. But I digress.

We'd have to be very desperate indeed to eat grass seeds, so they were unlikely to be a big part of the Palaeolithic diet. The invention of agriculture meant that we became more and more dependent on those grass seeds (grains) for more and more of our calories. Now just eight grain crops (wheat, corn, rice, barley, sorghum, oats, rye and millet) supply almost 60 per cent of the calories and half the protein consumed on earth. In short, the one thing that allowed us to dominate the planet also significantly narrowed the variety in our diet. The big question is, does that matter? We certainly didn't evolve in an environment where grains supplied a significant percentage of our protein or calories, but there's little doubt that there were Palaeolithic tribes whose diet included carbohydrates, protein and fat in modern proportions, albeit from vegetables, nuts and meat rather than grains. Humans are opportunistic omnivores. If it's edible and we're hungry, we can and will eat it. This means that our digestive system and metabolism are superbly adapted to enormous swings in the amounts of carbohydrates, fats and protein we consume. We'll make do with whatever we get. Better than that, we're good enough to thrive in just about any food scenario nature can throw at us, given enough time for evolution to work its magic.

Fructose and polyunsaturated fats are very specific substances that we have to extract industrially to consume in any great quantity. They are therefore substances with which we have absolutely no evolutionary experience (at least in the quantities to which we've been exposed in the last 200 years), whereas protein and glucose (the primary constituents of grains) are the stuff we grew up on (in an evolutionary sense). It's true we have no evolutionary experience of using grains to create food, but once it's eaten, the functional components (as far as our metabolism is concerned) are the same as those of the diet we evolved to eat.

Do grains make us fat and sick?

Societies with a diet of processed food eat less (and fewer) grains than societies that don't. They also eat less grains than their ancestors did before the advent of processed food. That's right, I said they eat *less* grains. According to the Reserve Bank of Australia's analysis of United Nations data, as a society becomes wealthier, it eats more sugar, more meat and less grains. And that

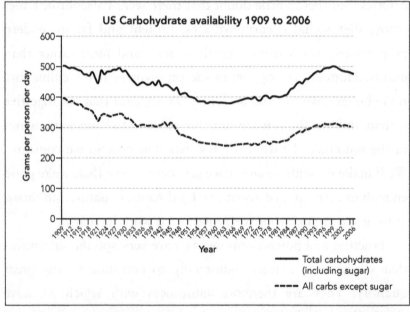

Americans now eat 25 per cent *less* non-sugar-based carbohydrates (largely grain and potato-based food) than at any time since 1909 (when such things started being recorded with precision). The latest upward bounce in the curve is the effect of the 'eat less fat and more carbs' dietary advice we've been given for the last three decades. The overall trend towards less carbs matches UN data, which confirms that as a society becomes more Westernised, it tends to eat less grain.

makes sense. Grains are cheap food. Rich people would rather buy a steak than eat bread (again).

Because per capita grain consumption decreased during the same time frame that modern chronic diseases increased, it seems highly unlikely that grain-based carbohydrates could be responsible for the rise in those chronic diseases. That's not to say they're completely exonerated.

It's clearly the case that fructose damages our ability to metabolise carbohydrates properly. Insulin is an important appetite-control signal generated in response to eating any carbohydrate (except fructose). Fructose affects the sensitivity of cells to that signal and degrades our ability to use carbohydrates for energy. The result is that those carbohydrates (whether they be from grains or vegetables) accumulate as fat and leave us with permanently raised blood sugar levels. So yes, carbs make us fat (and give us type 2 diabetes), but only because fructose has damaged the system that's supposed to stop that happening.

Cutting out carbs but continuing to eat fructose will not result in permanent weight loss or reversal of type 2 diabetes. So, for example, a 'Paleo' diet that avoids breads and other grains but still allows you to make desserts from dates (34 per cent fructose), honey (40 per cent fructose) or agave syrup (90 per cent fructose) is not really solving any problem. Cutting out fructose will, though, whether you eat carbs or not. If you want the weight loss or disease reversal to go faster in the beginning (we're all in a hurry), then cutting out carbs will certainly help while your appetite-control system is repairing itself. But non-fructose carbs are not likely to be the cause of modern disease. They're not the murderer, they're just the bloke who happened to find the body and was found (in)conveniently next to it when the police turned up.

Equally, there's nothing wrong with choosing to live without grains (or milk or both). Our species has certainly managed that for longer than any of us is likely to live. We just need to be sure we don't leap out of the dietary frying pan and into the fire. Replacing wheat flour with almond (or any nut) flour is not a good idea if you care how much omega-6 you consume (and you should). It's the dietary equivalent of replacing butter with margarine. Replacing cheese with 'cashew cheese' (it's a real thing – suggested for 'cheese'-cake) is even worse. And replacing cow's milk with almond milk is also not a good idea for exactly the same reason. Be sure that if you plan to eat like pre-agricultural man, the things you're eating are likely to be things you could pick off a bush, dig out of the ground or kill on the hunt. Believe me, cashew-cheese-cakes, agave syrup non-wheat brownies and almond milk were thin on the ground in the Palaeolithic period, so be careful.

What we eat really matters. I mean it *really* matters. You're driving a machine highly adapted to its environment. Don't lightly delete or add to its fuel source without understanding the biochemistry of what you're doing. The consequences can be significant and the cascades within our body can be catastrophic. This book suggests only two things: delete two dangerous items added to our diet in the last 200 years (sugar and seed oils) and otherwise Eat Real Food. Eating is not a hobby or an outlet for gastronomic creativity. It's a way of taking on fuel. This doesn't mean it has to be boring or tasteless, but it does mean you shouldn't mess with the fuel mix that the machine (your body) is adapted to consume.

Does the glycemic index (GI) of a food matter?

Because people are convinced that carbohydrates (rather than just fructose) are the cause of obesity, diets that restrict carbohydrates in general have become very popular. But low-carb diets can be a bit tricky to stick to if you're used to things like potatoes, bread, pasta, rice or pastry of any kind. Even a sausage roll is a quarter carbs. So in the spirit of making low-carbing easier, some enterprising folks have come up with a low-carb diet you can have if you'd really like to keep eating carbs. It's called the low-GI (for low–glycemic index) diet.

When we eat most carbohydrates (except fructose), they're slowly converted into our primary fuel – glucose – circulating in our bloodstream. Some foods are converted to glucose quickly and some do it more slowly. The same amount of glucose enters our blood either way; GI is just about timing. The theory behind GI is that foods that do it more quickly are in some way worse for us than foods that do it more slowly. So the promoters of this kind of diet spend most of their time measuring how fast carbohydrates in various foods are converted to blood glucose.

What is the GI?

Measuring GI is not an exact science. We all react differently to different foods and even the same person might react differently to the same food on different days. So at best the GI number is an average guess that might tell you (relatively speaking) how quickly a given food might be metabolised. And there's one aspect that makes it particularly unhelpful. GI is measured using a 50-gram sample of just the food being tested (50 grams of white bread, for example). But very few of us eat food that way. We eat our bread wrapped around a bacon and egg sarnie or we eat our potatoes with steak and three veg. All of these extra foods will dramatically affect how quickly we process the carbohydrate component of our meal. We have no way of knowing what the GI of those combinations might be without explicitly testing all of them (assuming we decided it was important to know).

So the calculations themselves have so many caveats as to render them almost completely useless as an estimate of how your body might react to a given food. That might be irrelevant if the outcome of eating this way were massive weight loss. Unfortunately, the news on that front is, well, disappointing (if you're trying to flog low-GI diets). Recent studies have confirmed what dieters have known for decades: low-GI diets work just as well (which is not really very well at all) as a low-calorie diet. And one very recent study has found that even people with type 2 diabetes, the group you would expect to do the best on a low-GI diet (because they're more sensitive to sharp rises in blood glucose), didn't do as well as type 2 diabetes sufferers placed on a high-GI diet.

The dangers of GI

Okay, so GI is useless, but it's not harmless. There is a fructose-sized loophole in the GI methodology large enough to drive a truck full of corporate exploitation straight through. Because our pancreas doesn't detect or respond to fructose (remember, glucose is our primary fuel, so we have no need of fructose detectors), it has an extremely low GI. Any food that contains fructose, either in its pure form or as part of sugar (sucrose), will therefore come up with an extremely low GI reading. Junk-food manufacturers figured this out very early on, which is why you'll see chocolate iceblocks, chocolate spread, chocolate milk flavouring and even bags of sugar labelled low-GI. All a food manufacturer need do is make sure they've loaded their product up with as much sugar as it can stand and Bob's your uncle, they have an instant health status that can be proudly plastered all over their sugar-filled junk food.

This significant and easily exploited loophole means anyone who blindly follows a low-GI diet that includes processed food is likely to cause long-term harm and make any insulin dependence worse over time. Low-GI diets are based on a false premise (that it matters how long it takes carbohydrates to be converted to glucose in the bloodstream) and are extraordinarily difficult to measure accurately anyway. But even if neither of those things mattered, the dangerous fructose blind spot takes them from the realm of dietetic nonsense into actively harmful to the people they should be helping. We should avoid low-GI diets at all costs.

Beware false prophets of health bearing superfoods

Even a cursory glance at the pages to this point should convince you we're in the midst of a chronic-disease epidemic. Rates of fatty liver disease, kidney disease, type 2 diabetes, cancer and heart disease (to name just a few) are increasing exponentially. The sicker we've become, the more we've sought to self-medicate. That's an environment ripe for exploitation by health gurus. Most are well meaning but they all have a certain modus operandi in common.

Because we're generally getting sicker despite doing exactly what the health establishment tells us to do, we're fertile ground

Super food	The claims	What the research says
Acai: berry from a South American palm	Lowers cholesterol, speeds up weight loss, and helps with arthritis symptoms	There are no independent (not sponsored by the people flogging acai) studies that support any of these claims
Activated almonds: almonds that are soaked	Soaking the almonds makes it easier for our body to access the nutrients	Soaking does break down some starches and proteins, but there's no evidence of that having any benefit in humans (beyond what would be obtained by eating unsoaked almonds)
Chia seeds: seeds from a form of mint that grows in Mexican deserts	Lowers cholesterol, triglycerides and blood pressure	There's no evidence of any of these claims being true, but chia seeds do have more omega-3 than most other seeds and so, with flaxseeds, are a better choice than most other seeds (if you really feel you need to eat seeds at all)
Chlorophyll: the green pigment from leaves, including grasses	Boosts energy and wellbeing	Eat anything green (except jelly babies) and you'll get all the chlorophyll you need (assuming you need any)
Coconut oil: oil extracted from coconuts (by crushing)	Weight-loss aid, improves Alzheimer's symptoms and general health and wellbeing	Coconut oil is a good fat because it's high in saturated fatty acids, but the observed benefits could be obtained from any fat or oil high in saturated fats (such as animal fat) as part of a low-sugar diet
Coconut water: coconut juice	Rehydration and a good source of minerals	Like any juice, the primary ingredient is sugar and there's no evidence we're deficient in any of the other trace minerals likely to be present. Water is a better choice for rehydration
Goji berries: Chinese berry	Usually marketed as a weight-loss aid or for their antioxidant properties	There's no evidence to support the claims. As far as antioxidants go (even assuming we can absorb them appropriately), a peek at the chart below should convince you they're nothing to write home about

for the suggestions of these false prophets of health. The number of us taking vitamin and mineral supplements has risen dramatically in the last three decades. Approximately half of all US adults and more than 63 per cent of those over 60 regularly take supplements. And the numbers are very similar in Australia, with around 43 per cent of all adults regularly using supplements. In the year 2000, Australians spent $1.67 billion on dietary supplements. This was four times the amount we spent on prescription drugs and triple the amount we spent just seven years earlier. As our health problems get worse and worse, we increasingly turn to over-the-counter supplements as part of the solution. We want a pill we can pop that makes us think we feel less lethargic or less stressed, or that makes our children smarter or our bones less brittle. And the supplements industry is only too happy to assure us they have the answer to all that and much more. Unfortunately, almost all supplements are completely unnecessary, and overconsumption of some can have disastrous outcomes. I've written about the perils of supplements in detail in *Big Fat Lies*.

That desire to fix ourselves has not only spawned a multibillion-dollar supplements industry, it has created a whole new category of food – the superfood. Superfood is a word made up by the false health prophets to flog us unusual foods at extraordinary prices. The reason we're supposed to be happy to part with a king's ransom for a hand-polished chia seed (not a real thing – I hope) is that it contains extraordinarily large amounts of some terribly important essential nutrient (that we've somehow been surviving without up to that point). Here's a sample of some of the recent substances marketed as superfoods. And just by way of comparison, I've mixed in some more common foods that in

many cases are significantly more potent (for what it's worth –
which is not much).

I'm sure there are many more 'superfoods' I haven't included
here, and more will be 'discovered' between when I write this and
when you read it, but there's just one thing you need to know about
superfoods. You don't need them. No human ever has. If you eat a
diet consisting of real food, you don't need any extra anything. You
don't need extra vitamins, extra minerals, extra fish oil (or krill oil)
or extra antioxidants. The human body evolved on a diet of real
food. It's perfectly adapted to extract exactly what it needs from
real food. Supplements (as pills or superfoods) are not required.
Don't fall for the false health prophets. Waste neither your time nor
your money on their insanely particular prescriptions for 'wellness'.
You'll be perfectly healthy just eating meat and three veg (and all
the other types of real food). Oh, and the next time someone tries
to tell you to eat goji berries, tell them to have a coffee instead.

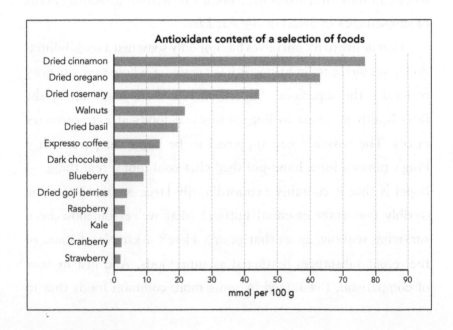

5

WHY DIETS (AND SURGERY) DON'T WORK

The diet industry wants us to believe that we gain weight because we're not good people. We suffer from a character defect. Well, two character defects, to be precise. We eat too much (the sin of gluttony) or we exercise too little (the sin of sloth) or usually both. If we're successfully convinced that our character defects are the source of our fatness, then the solution is clear. We must suffer for our sins and deprive ourselves. We must eat less and exercise more, banish the gluttony and sloth from our lives and once more return to the crowd of sin-free thin people.

Of course, there's no shortage of people lining up to tell us that their version of deprivation is more effective than the others, but empirically that can't be true. If any diet actually worked, it would quickly destroy the competition and eventually eliminate its own market. The world would be thin once again. Unfortunately, the sad reality of deprivation dieting is that it doesn't work. Or, to be more accurate, it does work for exactly as long as you're prepared to deprive yourself (which for most people is less than a year).

We like to save our brainpower for the hard decisions (like whether to order tea or coffee), so we run most of our body on autopilot. Temperature control, heartbeats, breathing – all are done automatically. We also run our digestive system on autopilot. It's perfectly capable of automatically determining exactly how much (and even what type of) food we need without us giving it a moment's thought. We can, however, override some of our automated systems. We can, for example, stop breathing. Try it now. See, that was easy, right? Trouble is, if you do that for even a few minutes, eventually your body will lose patience with your idiotic game and resume automatic control. Exactly the same thing happens when we choose to eat less by going on a diet. Consciously eating less food than our body thinks we need would be like choosing to take ten fewer breaths an hour. You can do it (if you're a good counter), but eventually your automated systems take over and restore your oxygen (and, in the case of diets, food) requirements. Attempting to use willpower to control automated processes is a fool's errand, but that's exactly what diet vendors ask people to do every single day of the week.

When we gain weight there'll be an accompanying increase in the amount of food we consume. It's just the same as when we exert ourselves. The harder we work, the more air we consume. No sane person would suggest that the increased airflow is what's making us exercise (if so, you'd do well to avoid standing near fans). It's obvious that the driving force in the exercise versus airflow equation is the exercise. The harder you work, the more air you consume. But when it comes to food, for some reason, nutritionists prefer a perverse view of the world. Their position is that increased food consumption causes the weight gain. In other words, we consciously choose to consume more food (implying some sort of character defect) and that drives weight gain. That's the equivalent of saying we choose to consume more air and that makes us do more exercise. Obviously, we breathe harder *because* we exercise and we eat harder *because* we need energy (or at least our body thinks it does). Not only is that logical, it doesn't require us to believe that overweight people suffer from a character defect.

We're perfectly happy to explain the equation that way when we talk about people (children) who grow vertically. But for some reason, when Norm grows horizontally, nutritionists magically reverse the cause and effect, lurching from physics to psychology – and the cause suddenly becomes Norm's gluttony or sloth (or both).

> **Eating is the way we put on weight, it isn't the reason we put on weight. Obesity is a symptom of dysfunction in our appetite-control hormones, not a character defect.**

Obesity is a symptom of a failure in the balance of hormones controlling how much food we take in. This hormone dysfunction causes us to store too much fat, but because our body isn't aware the fat is there, it keeps demanding food. Our body's response to insufficient food is to demand more, a response we know as hunger. When food isn't forthcoming, the body compensates by progressively shutting down energy-consuming systems and then using up muscle and protein (remember, it doesn't know the fat is available). Physical movement is minimised, sleep is the preferred option, body temperature is lowered and eventually even thinking (cognitive function uses a massive 25 per cent of the energy we consume) is minimised. None of these actions is a conscious decision. Our body's first line of defence to intentional deprivation is to ask for more food by making us feel hungry. Our ability to resist that signal varies enormously over time and depends a lot on our motivation and circumstances. When we ignore it, as we do with determination in the first few weeks of a diet, our body simply starts cutting down on energy consumption and, yes, losing weight (but not fat). But it will only do this for as long as we can resist our body's constant demand for food. Suggesting we can count calories makes the fundamentally flawed assumption that our body has a fixed calorie requirement and that all we have to do is feed it fewer calories than that.

Our appetite-control system thinks we're starving, even while we have more than enough fat packed away (usually in very unsightly places). When an obese person restricts the amount of food they eat by going on a diet, they're not changing the underlying dysfunction in their appetite-control system (unless they also eliminate all fructose). Their body thought it was starving before the diet, now it's really starving. It won't use its fat store to satisfy its need for food, because the hormonal disruption caused by fructose means it doesn't even know it's there. The hormones will force the body to sacrifice muscle and even organs to make up for the missing calories. And the whole time, the dieter will feel like they're starving to death. No wonder no one can stay on a diet!

How popular diets 'work'

With the exception of surgery (and I'll come to that), all weight-loss diets share two common themes: they require us to exercise our willpower (well, suffer, really – if you ain't suffering, it ain't a diet) and reduce the number of calories we consume. They all do it with loads of highly prescriptive rules to keep your mind off the fact you're starving, but none of them is any more sophisticated than that.

All diets work, but only for as long as we can use willpower to overcome hormones. Here's what the research says about some popular types of diets.

- **Meal-replacement shakes:** The recipe varies a little between brands (for example, The Biggest Loser, Betty Baxter, Optislim, Atkins Advantage, Herbalife) but the typical shake is one-third milk protein and almost half sugar, with just a smidgen of milk fat for taste (pretty much powdered milk plus sugar plus multivitamins). The research suggests an obese person can expect to lose 15–25 per cent of their body weight in the first six months of 'treatment', but after one year they'll have regained 16 per cent, after three years 18 per cent and after four years 20 per cent. For any other product that means outright failure, but for a diet those are pretty good results. The only problem is that those figures are only for the people who stick to the diet, and the research says they're the exception, not the rule. Almost half the participants drop out by the six-month mark. And even the iron-willed remainder start putting weight back on after those first six months.

- **Intermittent fasting (for example, the 5:2 Diet):** This type of diet typically cuts total calories by a quarter by allowing the dieter to eat normally five days a week and then severely restricting calories two days a week. It's a relatively recent type of diet so studies are limited, but one of the best so far concluded that after six months, the benefits of intermittent fasting were identical to those of a control group who just reduced calories by 25 per cent. Like all other willpower-based diets, adherence is the problem. By the end of that study, just 44 per cent of the intermittent fasters were still on the diet. At least it was better than the calorie-counters. Just 32 per cent of them were still going strong.

- **Low-carbing (for example, Paleo, Atkins, South Beach):** Studies of the effectiveness of low-carb diets generally reveal that the low-carbers end up eating the same number of calories as calorie-counters. Studies that have compared low-carbing to other forms of dieting (generally low-fat) find that people can stick to them more easily (as removing carbohydrates eliminates an important hunger signal and often incidentally removes sugar). After six months, low-carbers have generally lost twice as much weight as controls. Unfortunately, that's as good as the news gets. In general, the longer the study runs, the closer together the two groups get. By the twelve-month mark, those who are still complying have generally lost less than 5 per cent of their starting weight and are regaining it quickly. A very recent study obtained better results by working very hard to keep the participants on the diets. That resulted in just 20 per cent of them dropping out at the twelve-month stage and a slightly better weight-loss result for the low-carb followers at that point. Unfortunately, that study didn't account for the role that sugar (a carb) reduction played in the (twelve-month) positive result for the low-carb diet. Like other recent studies on low-fat and low-carb diets, the study confirmed that if people are actively reminded to keep exercising willpower, they can keep their appetite-control system at bay for longer.

- **Calorie-counting (for example, Weight Watchers, Lite n' Easy, Jenny Craig):** In 2007, Associate Professor Traci Mann and her colleagues from the University of California, Los Angeles (UCLA), analysed the outcomes of long-term randomised studies of calorie-restriction diets. They could find only seven sufficiently rigorous long-term studies that ran for two years or more. In those studies, the average weight loss at the end for the people on the diets was just 1.1 kilograms (and trending down), while the controls (those people not on any of the diets) gained 0.6 kilograms over the same period. Probably the best thing that could be said about all the diets studied was that they slowed the small weight gain that would otherwise have occurred. When dieters were followed for four or five years, their rate of weight gain didn't appear to level off in the way it did for non-dieters, suggesting that a diet puts a dint in a cycle of continuous weight gain but doesn't make any real long-term (greater than two-year) difference. Mann and her colleagues concluded that, statistically speaking, the best indicator that someone will be heavier in five years time is their being on a diet now.

Why diets *can't* work (if you keep eating fructose)

Diets ask us to fight an appetite-control dysfunction (caused by fructose) with willpower. Fighting automated appetite controls with willpower is about as effective as fighting the urge to breathe with willpower. We can expect early success, but eventually our body's in-built involuntary responses will win out. Diets don't and can't work because they don't affect the cause of weight gain.

On the other hand, fixing that dysfunction by removing fructose has almost magical effects. I deleted fructose from my diet ten years ago. I lost 40 kilograms in eighteen months without exercising one iota of willpower (other than breaking my addiction to fructose). But more importantly, my weight hasn't changed since. I've managed the impossible according to diet research. I've lost significant weight and kept it off in the long term. The research says that if I'd relied on willpower I'd now be at least as fat as I was before I cut sugar out. But I didn't need willpower. Deleting sugar cured the metabolic dysfunction that was causing me to be obese in the first place. I did it, thousands of people who've read *Sweet Poison* have done it and you can do it too – no willpower required.

Why weight-loss surgery changes nothing

When the diets inevitably fail, surgery becomes the last resort. Lap-band surgery is the most popular form of bariatric (obesity) surgery in Australia today. In 1993–94, just 550 lap-band procedures were performed in Australia, but by 2012–13 this had grown to 12,967, a whopping 24-fold increase in the market in less than two decades. This explosive growth has occurred even though Medicare rebates cover very little of the cost. Most people are paying the lion's share (around $13,000) themselves. And the expense doesn't stop there. Lap-banding is not a set-and-forget procedure. Constant surgery is required to adjust the device to find the sweet spot that allows people to control their appetite. In 2012–13, Australian doctors performed almost 111,000 of these adjustment operations.

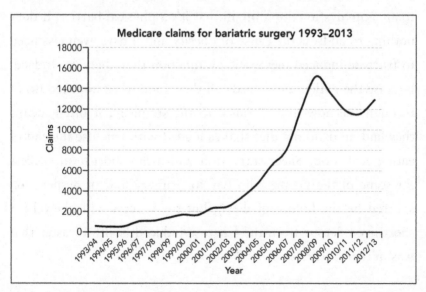

Lap-band surgery inserts an adjustable ring around the entry to the stomach. Keeping the ring tight ensures that very little can get into the stomach. It's a physical barrier for patients who are unable to overcome their apparent character defects with willpower alone.

But this invasive procedure is not a simple piece of cosmetic surgery. About one in five cases require a major re-operation, and for more than half of recipients, it doesn't result in any significant weight loss. Only two out of five will experience a remission in their type 2 diabetes (and then only for a maximum of nine years), and patients on average only gain an extra 1.2 years of life expectancy. Even worse, those appalling results are the outcomes from studies commissioned by the folks flogging the devices. We have no idea what those numbers would be in truly independent studies.

Lap-bands and other types of bariatric surgery are simply glorified versions of stitching people's lips together. It's a solution to appetite dysfunction only in that it's a physical barrier. It does nothing to address the cause of obesity and it pays even less heed to fructose-induced metabolic dysfunction than diets do. Indeed, because the patient now needs all their food to be liquefied (to fit through the now-tiny entrance to the stomach), it often means they end up drinking diet shakes loaded with fructose instead of eating real food. Sheer starvation will mean short-term success for some of the people who pay for surgery (out of desperation spurred by the failure of diets), but the success will likely be a short-lived detour from the fructose-induced health disaster that was in their future.

The food corporations are against you

If everything you've just read doesn't scare the gee willikers out of you, then you needn't read any further – you're already dead. Simply put, the science is increasingly homing in on one simple but unsurprising fact. When you expose an evolved machine (us) to unprecedented quantities of substances for which it has no adaptation, things break. This is especially true if one of these substances is our primary energy source (sugars) and the other is used in the construction of every cell in our body (polyunsaturated fats) – oh, and drives our immune system.

Very little of what I've set out to this point is new news in the research community. It's rare for it all to be put together in one place, but specialists in each area wouldn't be discovering anything new by reading the section that relates to their studies. The trouble is that most of them are paid to examine the bark on their particular scientific tree very closely. Almost none of them gets to see what the forest looks like from 30,000 feet. Sometimes that takes an outsider with no dog in the fight.

Even if researchers were inclined to gather the research from disparate fields together in one place and cross-analyse it, there are powerful forces working very hard to make sure that never happens. No, I haven't just reached for my tinfoil hat. There's no conspiracy at work. Those powerful forces are market forces, but these are not ordinary market forces – we've had those since the invention of money. No, the ones killing us all are those we've entrusted to psychopaths. No, still no tinfoil hat. Read on and I'll explain myself.

In 1855 we invented the limited liability corporation. A corporation is a made-up person with most of the legal rights of a person, but its only responsibility is to its shareholders. In almost all cases its purpose is to make more money for those shareholders. Everything else it does (except obey the laws of the land) comes second to that primary objective. Even if it does nice things like sponsor the local sports team, it does so because its shareholders are certain they'll make more money doing that than not. Corporations don't have morals or empathy. They have laws to obey and shareholders to please (by making money). This means that all corporations are essentially psychopathic in nature. Their profit tomorrow will always be more important than your health in twenty years (or anything else about you except how much money you can give to them now).

> 'Slavery is the legal fiction that a person is property. Corporate personhood is the legal fiction that property is a person.' – Anonymous

We've learnt this lesson over and over again, first with cigarette companies, then asbestos companies and then baby-formula companies using underhand tactics to dump product in Third World countries with filthy water supplies (where breastmilk is always the best option). But for some reason, we believe it will be different next time, even when some of those companies are the ones now stuffing us with fructose and seed oils. But let's be clear, they're not *trying* to hurt us, that's just an unfortunate (and not immediately profit-impacting, and therefore irrelevant) side effect.

The model is the same every time. An innovation leads to a product that's more addictive or cheaper to make than the competition. It doesn't appear to kill on contact (which would definitely hurt the marketing message), so it's rushed into production. It gives its inventor a lead on the market but eventually the whole market copies it. Long-term exposure to the substance (say, cigarette tar or asbestos or lead in petrol) eventually leads to scientists discovering chronic effects that weren't immediately apparent. But by then sales of the product have built multibillion-dollar corporations that are more than capable and more than willing (given their legally prescribed lack of empathy) to suppress the evidence, sponsor corruptible scientists to muddy the waters, and mount extensive lobbying and disinformation programs. This rarely defeats the truth, but it often squeezes an extra 50 years profit out of a substance that should have been removed from the shelves on the first day.

Most modern deaths are caused by diseases that barely affected anybody 200 years ago, and the science says that between them, sugar and seed oils are responsible for almost all of those deaths. The twin innovations of commercial sugar production (which made food addictive) and seed-oil manufacture (which made food cheap to make) have completely transformed our food supply in that time frame. At each turn, the corporations have successfully diverted attention away from their products as a possible cause. When sugar was first raised as a potential problem by John Yudkin in 1972, corporate power ensured those sponsoring a message friendlier to their interests prevailed. When WHO (the World Health Organization) again tried to make a move on sugar in 2003, corporate power threatened it with annihilation. The only reason it still exists is that it caved in to the threats. And when I first publicly raised concerns about seed-oil use in Australia in my book *Big Fat Lies*, powerful corporations publicly railed against both me and the message.

But expensive public-relations campaigns can't change the cold hard facts. Between 1980 and 2000, the number of us who were obese more than doubled. Between 1990 and 2005, the number of Australians with diagnosed type 2 diabetes also more than doubled. Between 1985 and 2000, the rate of new prostate cancers increased by 15 per cent a year, breast cancer by 37 per cent, and melanoma by 60 per cent in men and 22 per cent in women. There's only one possible explanation for why things have got so much worse in a period when we've been more conscientious about our health than ever before – the advice is wrong.

The obvious question is why the status quo isn't being questioned by the people who should have our best interests at heart. None of the research I've mentioned in this book is secret. Most of it is recent and very little of it is controversial. So why isn't it causing consternation and soul-searching among those in the nutrition and heart-health communities?

The sad reality is that there are very few groups of people or individuals whose role is to communicate developments in our knowledge of disease prevention. The Australian Heart Foundation receives sponsorship and endorsement fees from the processed-food industry and is especially prominent in promoting the consumption of margarine. The Dietitians Association of Australia is also heavily sponsored by the processed food industry. Together, these two groups are responsible for a significant percentage of the dissemination of 'healthy eating' information in this country. And while I'm not for a minute suggesting that they purposely set out to further their sponsors' interests, an obvious conflict of interest is inherent in the relationship.

Doctors don't suffer from a similar problem with the processed-food industry, and that may well be because they don't see advice about diet as part of their job. They're paid to fix things that are broken. For most doctors, the extent of dietary advice is to refer the patient to a dietitian. Medical researchers are equally unconcerned about diet. They're paid to find tools to sell to doctors (usually drugs) to fix things that are broken. Meanwhile, this constant research into 'cures' leads us into the false belief that we don't know much about what causes disease (how many times have you heard that we don't know what causes cancer?). And while that's clearly untrue, no one with a financial incentive will tell you otherwise. No one makes serious money telling you not to eat sugar or seed oils. Indeed, it's quite the opposite. There's much more money to be made in making sure you keep eating them.

But in the dark clouds of psychopathic (for want of a better term) corporate self-interest and conflicted defenders of our interest, there is a silver lining. None of them can get you if you just Eat Real Food. Knowledge is your friend. You don't need gatekeepers to tell you what you should or shouldn't eat. You're quite capable of finding out for yourself by reading books like this, or, if you prefer original evidence, by reading past what I say to the sources at the end of the book. Once you understand what real food is and why you should eat it, then no amount of corporate chicanery can take your health away or stop you healing. You are in control and guess what – your interests, rather than someone else's profit, become the priority.

You should also understand, however, that if you choose not to act to protect yourself, then the science says your chances of developing one of the awful diseases mentioned above are increasing by the day. We are the subjects of one of the most appalling experiments in human health manipulation ever conceived. The consequences of consuming ever larger quantities of fructose and omega-6 fats will make the damage inflicted by cigarettes and asbestos look like a paper cut. Even if you think I'm a certified nutbag, make sure you read the papers cited in the notes section, as well as the papers they cite. This is not fad-diet nonsense. It's very real and very dangerous and very few of us (or our kids) will live lives unaffected by sugar or seed oils unless we act now.

Why eating real food isn't a diet or a fad

Diets don't work. Well, they do, but only for as long as you can fight appetite-control dysfunction with willpower or surgery. And it doesn't matter how you do the dieting, whether you cut the carbs, cut the fat, count the calories or wolf down superfoods, they're all an exercise in futility. The reason is quite simple: compliance. We can only do mind over matter for just so long. We can only isolate ourselves from our friends and family, we can only afford weird and wonderful ingredients, we can only obsess about the exact number of grams or calories for just so long. Dieting is just not fun. And when we combine 'not fun' with 'focused willpower exertion 24/7', we get something that only the very rarest of Zen beings can manage for any reasonable duration and that nobody can manage for the rest of their life. Eating well is not meant to be hard work. It's not meant to be an obsession. It's not meant to be an exercise in complexity or expense. It's meant to be an enjoyable and effortless way to fuel our lives for the rest of our lives.

Eating real food delivers on those aims. By removing the addictive and dangerous elements added by the profiteers, it takes us back to the basics of eating in a way we can not only manage but also enjoy – forever. Eating real food works because it:

- doesn't involve willpower
- is inexpensive and time-efficient
- is based on readily available ingredients
- draws on all food groups
- allows you to make quick purchase decisions once you know the rules (no standing paralysed by indecision in the health-food section of Coles)
- has a few logical and simple – though very important – restrictions
- quickly becomes a way of life
- allows you to travel, go to restaurants and feed your kids (without endangering their lives or health).

But this isn't just about weight loss. As it turns out, for most people, eating real food will result in weight loss (if they need to lose weight). But even if we didn't lose a gram, I'd still be strongly advocating you do it. If you do, you'll avoid the fructose and polyunsaturated fats that have been dumped into your 'food' by psychopathic profiteers. And in so doing you'll take yourself and your kids off the spectrum of a host of very nasty chronic diseases.

Now you know why you need to Eat Real Food, let's get down to tin tacks. How? The rest of this book is devoted to answering that question. It's the modern human's practical guide to extracting real food from a machine designed to produce nothing but fake food. You won't find arbitrary and unjustifiable rules. I won't be telling you what you must eat, just how to avoid the two things you must avoid: sugar and seed oils. Beyond that, it's entirely up to you. If you like meat, then eat meat. If you don't, then don't. But in each case I'll do my best to tell you what you'll miss out on and how you can compensate.

My recommendations are based on the science around what's in our foods, not on what's popular at the Paleo Café or in this year's best-selling detox diet. I won't be asking you to buy coconut anything (unless you like coconuts). You won't find requests for other unusual or expensive ingredients either. I'll show you a simple yet delicious way to feed yourself in the safest possible way (according to the science). And I'll do my best to explain why. After you implement my real food plan, your food bills will decrease, your health will improve, and you'll know exactly what you and your family are eating and why. Attack!

Part Two

HOW TO EAT REAL FOOD

6

WHAT TO KEEP AND WHAT TO BUY

If you're reading this, then the first part of the book has done its job. It's convinced you that you and your family's life will be immeasurably better (and probably considerably longer) if you Eat Real Food. You'll have a reasonable chance of avoiding or reversing all of the chronic diseases I've listed and you'll be doing your absolute best to ensure your children and loved ones do, too. And all you'll need do is eat the way your great-grandparents did. Easy, right? Well, yes, but you need to go in with the right mindset. It sounds simple: all you do is buy whole food instead of packaged, processed fake food. But beneath that simple message lies some serious complexity in a society geared to making sure the last thing you do is Eat Real Food. You'll need to know how to shop, how to cook and when it's safe to take shortcuts. Oh, and just for good measure, while you're doing all that, you'll be dealing with breaking an addiction that's not too dissimilar to quitting smoking.

This part of the book is designed to be your best friend during the first few difficult months as you start out on your quest for real food. It's also meant to be a handy reference once you're in cruise mode. It will guide you through the supermarket, break that nasty little sugar addiction and even give you some pointers on how to cook with ingredients you've probably only heard about when the fossils talk about the good old days. Let's start with navigating the safe paths through the forest of fake food.

Losing the fake food

Before you can start eating real food you need to remove all the fake food from your life. This will involve some pain. Because sugar is a major ingredient in fake food and it's addictive, you'll probably be throwing out some of your best friends (we'll come to how to deal with that shortly). If you can't stand the waste, I'm sure you'll find a good home for most of it. Either have a last binge yourself (definitely not the preferred option, but hey, let's be realistic here) or donate the food to your fake-food-eating friends.

To help you out, I've prepared some lists of what you should keep or buy (real food) and what you should chuck or ignore (fake food).

If you think that looks like a shopping list from the 1800s, you're probably not far from the truth. That list is from a time before the food manufacturers took hold of our collective diets.

REAL FOOD (KEEP ALL OF THIS)

Good sweeteners (see 'Sweetener cheat sheet' below)

Meat, poultry and game

Seafood

Eggs

Flour

Unsweetened breakfast cereals

Whole fruit and berries

Whole legumes, nuts and seeds

Whole vegetables

Butter

Unsweetened cream

Unsweetened milk

Cheese

Unsweetened (natural or Greek) yoghurt

Tea and coffee

Unflavoured water

Spirits

Beer

Dry wine

Good fats (see 'Fats and oils cheat sheet' below)

It's from a time when most people made most of what they ate from scratch and food was a pretty simple affair. That largely homemade food fulfilled a pretty simple function: it kept us alive and it didn't create chronic disease.

Now that you know what you definitely need to keep, here's a list of what you definitely need to get rid of. You don't need to read labels, you don't need fancy calculators – if it's on this list, it's gone. The fake-food list includes many things we've been told are healthy, but you need to put that out of your mind and move them all out of your life. If it helps, think of all the diseases you'll be avoiding just by doing this one simple dump run. Of course, this also means you'll never be buying any of this stuff again.

FAKE FOOD (DITCH ALL OF THIS)

Bad sweeteners (see 'Sweetener cheat sheet' below)

Marinated meat

Dried fruit

Margarine

Soft drinks

Fruit juice

Vegetable juice

Sweetened breakfast cereals

Jams, preserves and honey

Sweetened cream

Sweetened milk

Tomato and barbecue sauce

Cakes and sweet biscuits

Confectionery (yes, including chocolate)

Ice-cream

Sweetened yoghurt

Flavoured water

Pre-mixed spirits

Ciders (alcoholic and non-alcoholic)

Sweet-tasting wines

Bad fats (see 'Fats and oils cheat sheet' below)

I didn't want to clutter up the lists with detailed lists of sweeteners, fats and oils, but you do need to be able to tell the good from the bad. The cheat sheets below sort it out for you.

There are three categories of sweetener: those that are absolutely safe to consume, those that may be safe in limited doses, and those that aren't safe under any circumstances (usually because they're metabolised to fructose anyway).

The 'Your call' sweeteners are often several hundred to several thousand times sweeter than sugar. They're on that list because there's no reliable science suggesting they're dangerous, but they're all relatively new additions to our diet. It's been 200 years since we introduced sugar into our diet in significant quantities, and the science is only now showing the harmful effects. Ask me in

Sweetener cheat sheet

Not bad	Your call	Bad
Glucose (may be labelled as Corn Syrup, Dextrose or Glucose Syrup) Lactose Maltose Maltodextrin Maltodextrose Rice malt syrup	Acesulfame potassium (950) Alitame (956) Aspartame (951) Aspartame-acesulfame (962) Cyclamates (952) Erythritol (968) Neotame (961) Saccharin (954) Stevia (960) Sucralose (955) Xylitol (967)	Agave syrup Fructose Fruit juice extract Golden syrup High-fructose corn syrup (HFCS) Honey Inulin Isomalt (953) Lactitol (966) Litesse Maltitol (965) Mannitol (421) Maple syrup Molasses Polydextrose Resistant (malto)dextrin Sorbitol (420) Sucrose (sugar) Wheat dextrin

200 years if those sweeteners are fine. For now I'd try to avoid them or treat them as methadone for sugar addicts (use them to get off the gear but don't plan on using them in the long term). If you're interested in a detailed analysis of the science around each of these sweeteners, then take a look at *The Sweet Poison Quit Plan*. Notice that none of those on the good list has a number, so if you see numbers on a label, it's either bad or dubious.

The sweet recipes in Chapter 10 of this book all use one or more of dextrose, glucose syrup or rice malt syrup (all on the not bad list). All of these sweeteners contain no fructose, the addictive and damaging half of sugar. This of course means your cakes and bickies will no longer have that addictive quality, but that's the price you'll pay for your new slim and healthy body.

Fats and oils cheat sheet

Good	Use with caution (if at all)	Bad
Olive	Hazelnut	Canola (rapeseed)
Coconut	Cashew	Sunflower
Avocado	Almond	Safflower
Sustainable palm and	Peanut	Soybean (soy)
palm kernel	Pistachio	Rice bran
High-oleic sunflower (see	Flaxseed (linseed)	Corn
page 164)		Grapeseed
Macadamia		Cottonseed
Chestnut		Sesame seed
Butter		Pumpkin seed
Ghee		Other nut oils (including
Animal fat (includes lard,		walnut, pecan, pine,
tallow, fowl fat, etc.)		Brazil, etc.)

The criterion for which column above an oil or fat appears in is the amount of omega-6 fat the substance contains. The oils in the middle are rated 'Use with caution' largely because they contain borderline large-ish amounts of omega-6. This means that if one of these oils is a staple in your daily cooking, you should consider switching to one from the good list, but if you use them only occasionally, they're fine to keep.

UNDERSTANDING OIL LABELLING

There's no regulation of claims made on bottles of oil in Australia, so producers really can say what they like. There is, however, a voluntary code for olive-oil producers in line with international standards. Here's what the labels should mean:

Virgin: means that no heat or chemicals have been used to extract the oil from the fruit. A 'virgin' olive oil has a free-fatty-acid content (a measure of quality where lower is better – see 'Cooking fats' on page 204) that is less than 2 per cent. A 'virgin' coconut oil should have a free-fatty-acid content less than 0.5 per cent. Ninety per cent of the world's coconut-oil producers have agreed to adhere to this standard.

Extra virgin: An extra virgin olive oil has a free-fatty-acid content lower than 0.8 per cent. You might also see 'extra virgin' on a bottle of coconut oil, but there's no standard definition of that term for coconut oil, so it's probably best to treat it as 'virgin'.

Cold-pressed or first cold-pressing: means the oil was manually extracted without the use of chemicals or heat. Since this has to be the case to call it 'virgin', it's redundant labelling. There's no such thing as a 'second press' of an oil, so 'first press' is a meaningless addition to a redundant description.

Refined: means that the oil didn't make the cut as a 'virgin' because its free-fatty-acid content was too high or there were other impurities. It has been refined using chemical and physical filters to lower the free-fatty-acid content (to less than 0.3 per cent). Refined oil is pale and tasteless. It will be labelled 'pure', 'mild' or 'light' ('refined' is sure to put consumers off so it's rarely used on the label). This is a perfect choice as an ingredient where you want a vegetable-based fat but don't want the taste of olives or coconut in the final product. We use refined olive oil in our Mayonnaise recipe (see page 264).

Pure or no description: see 'Refined'.

Light or mild, or extra light or mild: see 'Refined'.

Whole foods

Not all meat is the same. Bacon from free-range pigs is much lower in bad fats than bacon from lot-fed pigs, because they don't eat anywhere near as much grain (which is relatively high in omega-6 polyunsaturated fats). Not all fruit is the same. Grapes, apples and bananas have much more sugar and much less fibre than almost any berry. This section is where we get down to the details. We look at what matters and what doesn't if you're going to get picky about food. If you're not a detail kind of person, then just copy the lists above and run with them. As long as what you're buying is whole or assembled food, you'll have eliminated 90 per cent of the potential harm. But if you're the kind of person who likes to understand the differences between the choices you have and (since you're spending the money anyway) make the best choice you can, then read on. Let's start with whole foods (the things that don't have labels).

Animal products

Real-food eaters want to minimise their total polyunsaturated-fat intake and also minimise the proportion of these fats that come from omega-6 fats. If you're eating ruminant animals (cattle and sheep), you don't need to worry too much whether it's lot-fed or not (although it would be nice if it weren't), but when it comes to omnivores (pigs, for instance) or seafood it matters a lot more. The sections below provide detailed guidance on what to look out for in the meat section.

Beef and milk

You are what you eat and if you eat meat, you are what it ate too, so it's good to know what that was. Cattle don't naturally eat grain. They have a decided preference for grass, but because cattle fed grain tend to fatten up faster, they're increasingly being raised on grain (for the final months of their lives) rather than grass. It's a lot more economical (because you can run a lot more cattle per hectare) to keep cattle in pens and feed them bulk grains, and so that's increasingly what the profit-driven providers of our food do.

DOES IT MATTER WHAT OUR CATTLE EAT?

Just as it does with us, a high-grain diet increases the proportion of omega-6 fatty acids in body fat (and milk).

Grain-fed beef has an omega-6 to omega-3 ratio of 15:1 compared with the grass-fed ratio of about 2:1.

But because cattle are ruminants (mammals with an ability to ferment grasses to produce nutrients), their gut removes any excess polyunsaturated fats, so the total polyunsaturated-fat content of their meat is the same whether they're grass-fed or grain-fed. But grains contain almost no omega-3 fats. So, while obviously it is preferable for beef to be grass-fed (because the ratio of omega-6 to omega-3 is much better), it shouldn't be a deal breaker if it's not, because the absolute levels of polyunsaturated fat in beef are still quite low.

In Australia today, all beef cattle start on pasture. They begin life on their mother's milk, and are weaned from pasture-based breeding cows between the ages of four and nine months. They're then 'backgrounded' on pasture until they're twelve to eighteen months old. Then they're generally sold to either a grass- or grain-finisher (feedlot) where they'll spend the last two to four months of their lives. In that time, they can be expected to put on the final third of their body weight (at the rate of 1.5 kilograms a day). Grass-finishing to the same weight takes about 50 per cent longer, which is why it's a less economically popular option.

UNDERSTANDING BEEF LABELS

There are no regulations governing the claims made about a beef animal's diet in Australia, but here's a guide to what they're trying to convey on the label.

Grass-fed: This should mean the animal has lived on a diet of grass its entire life, but since there are no labelling rules in Australia governing the use of this term, you just have to trust that they're being honest.

Grain-fed: This means that the animal was fed grain towards the end of its life and that about a third of its body weight comes from grain.

Grass-finished: See 'Grass-fed'.

Grain-finished: See 'Grain-fed'.

Organic: As there are no Australian rules governing the use of this term, it means whatever they want you to think it means. It doesn't necessarily mean the animal was grass-fed.

Certified organic: Finally, something a little bit enforceable – this means the organic claim has undergone a verification process that's laid out in an Australian standard. It still doesn't necessarily mean the cattle were grass-fed.

Pasture-raised: All cattle are raised on pasture for some part of their life. The term is meaningless.

Wagyu and **Angus:** Both these (expensive) types of beef are grain-fed.

Most of the beef (around 80 per cent) sold in Australian supermarkets is now grain-fed. It won't be labelled grain-fed – in fact, the label will tell you exactly nothing about what the animal ate. But here's a pro-tip. The fat on grain-fed beef tends to be white, whereas the fat on grass-fed beef is more yellow-ish. Take a close look at the meat next time you're in the supermarket, and chances are you'll be able to pick up some grass-fed beef without the fancy labelling and the premium prices that often go with it.

But don't sweat it too much. Australian grain-fed beef contains only about 0.5 gram more omega-6 per 100 grams than grass-fed beef. Just avoid the seed oils everywhere else in your diet and you'll be fine.

Milk is a similar story. Humans who eat diets high in seed oils have breastmilk high in omega-6 fats and the same goes for all other mammals and their milk, including dairy cows. But we're safe for now. So far there are very few feedlot dairies in Australia.

Lamb

About two in five Australian lambs are lot-fed for the last half of their lives (about eight weeks). Just as with cattle, a higher proportion of the fat in these lambs will be omega-6 than in lambs that have been entirely pasture-raised, but in the context of a real food diet, the difference will be insignificant. Australian lamb contains in total about 1 gram of omega-6 fat per 100 grams.

As with beef, if your budget can stretch to it, grass-fed lamb is a better option, but once again, don't worry too much about it.

Eggs and chicken

Chickens are birds that eat grain. But the science has now established conclusively that the exact mix of grain makes an enormous difference to the omega-6 fat content of chicken meat and eggs. Meat and eggs from chickens fed the commercial mix of corn and soybean meal used in the United States have twice the concentrations of omega-6 fats as products from chickens fed the mixture more likely to be used in Australia (barley, wheat and sorghum meal). US studies have shown that as a result of that higher omega-6 content, humans consuming diets containing those eggs have significantly higher LDL cholesterol oxidation rates (see Chapter 3 for why this matters).

ARE EGGS BAD FOR YOU? SHORT ANSWER: NO

If you were limited to eating just one food then your best bet would be eggs. They contain everything we need in roughly the right proportions. But that didn't stop health authorities vilifying them in the 1990s because of their cholesterol content.

We were told to avoid eggs and especially egg yolks (which kicked off a craze for egg-white omelettes).

But by 1999, studies were starting to suggest that there's absolutely no association between egg consumption and our chances of developing heart disease (despite eggs being quite high in cholesterol – which is yet another reason to discount that particular theory of heart disease).

Interestingly, a 2006 review of studies on the potential danger of eggs concluded that eggs seem to be one of the few things (besides deleting sugar or eating more saturated fat) that will convert a person from pattern B (heart attack waiting to happen) to pattern A (a picture of rude heart health; see Chapter 2). Ironically the Heart Foundation had been warning us not to consume the very thing that would ensure we weren't candidates for heart disease.

Australian chooks primarily eat wheat and sorghum, so for once economics (those are the cheapest grains here) are accidentally on the side of good health. Eggs and chicken aren't totally free of polyunsaturated fats, so it's probably not a good idea to switch to an 'all-egg' diet, but at the levels most people are likely to consume them, they're not of any great concern. Even more importantly, eggs contain a large range of highly beneficial nutrients that few other foods (except liver) can match.

> **Even if you ate four eggs a day, you'd only just be starting to exceed your allowance of omega-6 fats, so have an egg on that (homemade) toast.**

Bacon and pork

Beef and lamb are grain-fed, but it doesn't significantly increase the omega-6 fat content of the final product. Australian chickens are (luckily) fed the right grains. But when it comes to pigs we're straying into dangerous territory for the real-food consumer. Pigs are omnivores like us. They have no upper limit on the amount of omega-6 they'll store in their fat and they'll keep every bit of it they're ever given. And unlike cattle, pigs are grain-fed for their

---

IS YOUR PORK REALLY FREE-RANGE?

A free-range pig gets about two-thirds of its food from foraging in pasture, and relies on humans for fruit, vegetables, dairy products and grains. Only Australian pork labelled 'Australian Certified Organic', 'Demeter' (Bio-Dynamic Research Institute) or 'Humane Choice' is likely to be genuinely free-range.

entire life (after being weaned from a grain-fed mother). If the pigs producing your meat were lot-fed (as 94 per cent of Australian pigs are), then their fat will be higher in omega-6.

If you choose to eat full-fat lot-fed bacon, five slices will dispose of your entire daily allowance of omega-6 fat. If bacon is your thing, then it's better to go for rashers that have the fat trimmed off. See, it *is* possible for me to agree with the Heart Foundation. Around here, we like our bacon with all the fat but we don't have it that often (maybe once a week and then really a maximum of two rashers per person). A better everyday breakfast meat is beef (we have it in the form of sausages). Two middle rashers of full-fat bacon weigh about the same as one and a half beef sausages but

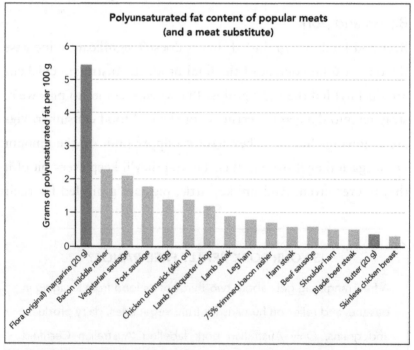

Trimmed bacon is a better choice when your bacon comes from grain-fed pigs (as almost all pork products in Australia do). The margarine and butter are just there for a sense of scale.

have four times the polyunsaturated-fat content. I've set out the relative polyunsaturated-fat contents in the graph above, and just for a sense of scale I've compared them to 20 grams each of butter and margarine (about the amount you might put on a couple of pieces of toast).

Vegetarian sausages aren't a great option either (because of their high soy content), so if you don't eat meat, mushrooms or lentils might be better choices.

Seafood

The perverted heart-health advice of the last half-century has driven a mass replacement of animal fats with man-made 'seed oils' (such as sunflower, canola and soybean). But it's also made us scared of red meat. We've been implored to eat more 'heart-healthy' fish instead. And we've listened. Since 1975, Australians have doubled their per capita consumption of fish.

The only way fish suppliers have been able to keep up with that kind of explosive demand is to invent a whole new industry: fish farming. And just like the cattle in feedlots, our farmed fish are increasingly being fed seeds, with devastating effects on their omega-3 levels.

Fish, being vertebrates just like us, are no more capable of making omega-3 fats than we are. Just like us, they need to get them from their diet. If they're carnivores (like salmon and barramundi), that means eating herbivorous fish that have been chowing down on seaweed high in omega-3. If the fish was wild-caught, it will have the expected supply of omega-3 on board. Nature's like that, it just works (as long as we leave it alone). If, however, the fish is farmed, then all bets are off.

The only way to ensure that farmed carnivorous fish get their omega-3s is to feed them oil from wild-caught fish (think of it as omega-3 capsules for fish). But it takes about 5 kilograms of wild-caught (but otherwise unsaleable) fish to produce 1 kilogram of farmed eating fish. In 1950 this wasn't a problem. There were barely any fish farms and there was an abundance of wild-caught fish. But now more than half of all fish consumed in Australia is farmed rather than wild.

In 2010, we maxed out the available supply of fish oil for farmed fish. But don't worry, the fish feeders have a solution – just mix in seed oil instead. Increasingly, fish feed is being created using the very same seed oils that now infest the remainder of our food supply. The Australian fish-farming industry now proudly boasts that it uses the lowest amount of fish oil in the world. It has replaced it with chicken fat and canola oil. The result is fish that are very high in omega-6 and very low in omega-3 (the very thing we've been advised to get by eating fish). When scientists have compared fillets from seed-oil-fed and fish-oil-fed fish, in general the amount of omega-3 has halved (and is sometimes considerably less) and the omega-6 fats have increased fivefold.

If you caught the fish yourself, you know it's wild-caught (obviously), but if you're relying on others, you're going to need to take their word for it. There are no labelling standards for farmed seafood in Australia. You'll need to keep an eagle eye out for the claims made on the pack in a supermarket or you'll need to develop a good relationship with your fishmonger. Fish farming is seen as the ecologically responsible thing to do (and it is, if we're to conserve wild fish stocks), so you'll see plenty of labels boasting the 'sustainability' of the fish. Unfortunately, this usually means it was farmed. If a fish is farmed (more than half are), avoid it unless you can be absolutely certain it hasn't been fed seed oils.

Of course, there's no need to seek out fish at all. Real-food eaters don't need to boost their omega-3 intake. And if we all ate a lot less fish, we'd simultaneously reduce the pressure on wild-caught fish and remove the economic incentive to farm them. Real-food eaters will easily get the 1.5 grams of omega-3 a day from everything else they eat – a couple of buttered cheese sandwiches would do it. But you just might like the taste and the variety. So if you do occasionally eat fish, it's wise to apply an omega-6 avoidance rule and go for the species that are lowest in omega-6 fats. To help you choose, the following chart gives the fat content of some of the seafood you're likely to encounter in Australia.

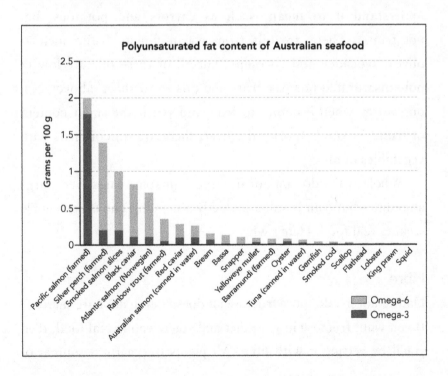

Based on the chart, you should be able to eat flathead, lobster, prawns and calamari (squid) without worrying about their omega-6 content. But as you move further to the left on the chart, be increasingly cautious. Bear in mind that an average serving of fish is 200–250 grams, so these numbers need to be at least doubled to show how much you'd be likely to consume in a single sitting.

Fruit

When it comes to fruit and veg, there's no need to be concerned about the fat content. Yes, seed oils are labelled as 'vegetable oils' but no vegetables were harmed during their construction. There's no such thing as oil from a vegetable ('vegetable' in this instance being simply used to indicate what we generally understand it to mean, such as carrots and potatoes, but not fruits). There are oils from warm-climate fruits such as olives, avocados and coconuts, but all of these oils are low in polyunsaturated fats (see 'Fats and oils cheat sheet' above). No, our worry when it comes to fruit and veg is the sugar content of fruit. As you'll shortly discover, there are no concerns with vegetables at all.

Whole fruits do contain fructose – in some cases, very large amounts – but fruit is still a perfectly acceptable choice for people seeking real food. Here's why.

Fibre

Nature doesn't do 'pure fructose'; it doesn't even do 'pure sucrose'. If you want fructose in your diet and you're eating real food, then you'll be getting it with fibre. All plants (the natural sources of fructose) contain fibre when served in their original packaging (and not juiced or otherwise manipulated to extract the sugar). Fibre slows down the absorption of fructose and gives our liver a fighting chance to deal with it properly. Studies show our digestive system can deal with the fructose in a couple of pieces of fruit when it comes with all the fibre intact, and that should come as no real surprise. Before the nineteenth century, that was pretty much the only way we'd be exposed to fructose anyway. At our place we always have some whole fruit on hand for when the kids get the munchies. Fruit really only becomes a problem if we strip out the fibre (by juicing). You'd need to juice three to four large apples to produce the juice in a small (250 millilitre) glass of juice. A child will easily drink a small glass of juice alongside a full meal. But try giving them four large apples and then expecting them to eat anything else. The juice and the apples contain the same amount of fructose, but one is a meal and one is an insignificant add-on to a meal.

> **Fruit juice is pure sugar and water, but the fruit it comes from contains the fibre antidote to the fructose poison it contains.**

The same goes for dried fruit (or congealed fruit juice, as I prefer to call it).

Water

The second feature of fruit that makes it safe is that it contains a lot of water, which, with the fibre, gives it bulk. That bulk significantly affects how much fructose we can take in from the fruit.

Drying the fruit has the same effect as juicing it: it concentrates the sugar and eliminates the bulk. With dried fruit, the fibre is still present, but the lack of bulk enables you to consume significantly larger quantities than if you were eating the whole fruit. A small box (40 grams) of sultanas contains all the sugar of about 130 grapes (approximately half a kilogram). You shouldn't eat either in one sitting, but it's very easy to do so with the handful of sultanas contained in the box.

How much fruit should we eat?

Whole fruit is a fine addition to any diet but the protection that fibre and water provide against the dangers of fructose only goes so far. Some of the most recent fibre research suggests that what's eaten with the fibre matters a lot. Soluble fibre eaten as part of whole grains drags through some of the starch for digestion as if it were fibre, but the effect is far less significant with fibre eaten as part of fruit. By increasing the proportion of fruit in your diet, you eliminate some of the other, starchier sources of carbohydrate, and reduce the overall beneficial effect of the fibre.

> It's perfectly acceptable to eat no fruit, but if you want to partake in nature's dessert buffet, it's a good idea to keep consumption under two pieces a day (for adults) or one piece a day (for children).

Which fruit should we eat?

Not all fruit is created equal. It's best to seek out fruit that's low in fructose and high in fibre, but some of the most popular fruits are just the opposite.

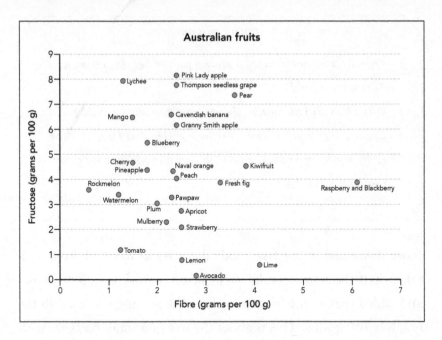

Australian fruits

The graph above shows a selection of fruits you're likely to find in the local supermarket. It plots each fruit's fibre content against its fructose content. The further towards the top-left corner of the graph (high-fructose, low-fibre) a fruit lies, the less desirable it is. Fruits in the bottom-right corner (low-fructose, high-fibre) are the best choice.

The amount of fructose in a given fruit differs between varieties. So, for example, some types of apple are much sweeter than others. Since the sweetness comes largely from fructose, this means that sweeter apples are higher in fructose. How ripe a piece of fruit is also changes the fructose content. As fruit ripens, it converts glucose to fructose. That's why ripe bananas taste sweeter than unripe ones. In the graph, I've used average amounts of fructose for each fruit type, just to give an idea of their relative positions.

Most fruits contain a mix of glucose, fructose and sucrose. To calculate the total fructose, I have looked up standard values (like

FRUIT RULES

- *Try not to consume more than two pieces per day for an adult or one for a child.*
- *Dried fruit and fruit juices should be completely avoided.*
- *Choose fruit that has lower fructose and higher fibre. Use the chart above as a rough guide. You want foods that are close to berries on the chart.*

those contained in my free foods database at davidgillespie.org), taken half the sucrose value (remember sucrose is half fructose) and added that to the fructose value. The serving size used in the graph is 100 grams. This is about the size of a small banana (with skin), a large banana (without skin) or a medium apple (with skin).

Fibre content varies significantly between fruits. So even though 100 grams of raspberries has the same amount of fructose as a navel orange, it's a better choice because it has more than twice the fibre. Strawberries and blackberries score well, too. The best fruit is passionfruit (not shown because it wrecks the graph – it has 14 grams of fibre and just 2.65 grams of fructose), but for those who prefer something a little less seedy, kiwifruit and fresh figs are good choices. At the other end of the scale, grapes and lychees are to be avoided, and caution needs to be exercised around apples, pears, bananas, mangoes, cherries, pineapples and apricots. Now you know why apple and grape purée is the filler of choice for a large proportion of fruit-based snacks. The manufacturers can claim these products have 'no added sugar' while they're actually serving up something very high in sugar (especially when puréed).

Vegetables

You can't go wrong with whole vegetables. Most contain fructose but nowhere near as much as fruit.

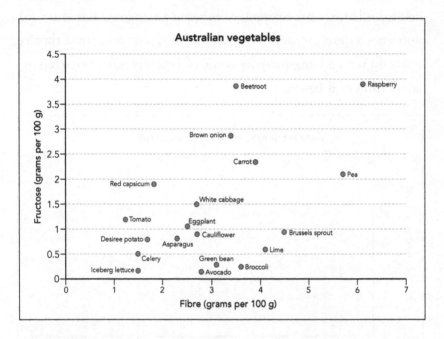

The graph above plots fructose against fibre for many of the vegetables you're likely to encounter in the supermarket. Note that the scales are not the same as in the fruit graph. The vegetable with the highest fructose content (beetroot) would be in the same position as the raspberry (one of the fruits with the lowest fructose content) in the fruit graph.

The serving size is once again 100 grams. That's approximately one small tomato, one medium onion. While none of the vegetables on the chart could be described as bad for you (in anything but humungous quantities), given the choice, go for broccoli, pumpkin, Brussels sprouts or beans ahead of carrots or peas.

Just in case vegetables aren't your favourite food in the whole world, you may be wondering if some are better for you than others, regardless of their sugar content. It's a question some quite helpful scientists have recently bothered to answer. Based on the nutrients (vitamins and minerals) each vegie contains, they've come up with a bang-for-buck scale of vegetables. I've charted my adaptation of it below.

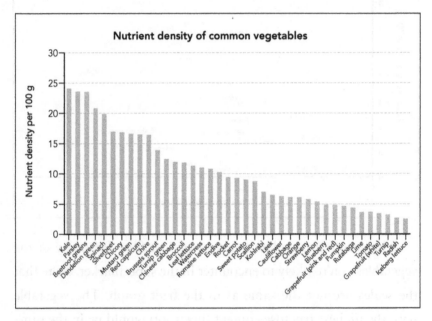

Spinach is indeed a good choice – looks like Popeye was right!

The numbers up the side have no practical meaning. The point of the graph is to show you how your favourite vegetable rates relative to other options. So if you're considering eating 100 grams of iceberg lettuce, a better choice would be 100 grams of parsley (not that I'd consider eating 100 grams of either, but you get the idea). Because animals concentrate nutrients, meats would often end up at the upper end of this scale (the left). But if you're avoiding meat, this will help you decide which vegies give you the most nutritional firepower.

The same warnings apply to vegetable juices as fruit juices. Juicing a vegetable is no better for you than juicing a fruit, because it simply extracts all the sugar and concentrates it. While carrot juice contains only half the sugar of apple juice, there's still the equivalent of two and a half teaspoons of the stuff in a small (250-millilitre) glass.

> On your shopping expedition, fill your
> basket with as much vegetable matter as
> you can stomach. You'll get well and truly
> sick of it long before it makes you sick.

Seeds and nuts

Obviously seeds (and nuts) contain seed oil. And, relative to any other real food you might be eating, it's quite a lot. This doesn't mean you need to avoid seeds and nuts completely, it just means you need to be careful about the quantities you consume. Extracting oil from seeds and nuts is the processed-food industry's version of juicing fruit. If you were to consume a cup (46 grams) of dried sunflower seeds you'd be taking in 10 grams of polyunsaturated oil (mostly omega-6). But a cup of sunflower oil would supply more than six times that much polyunsaturated fat (63 grams). Even so, the cup of sunflower seeds will have singlehandedly blown your omega-6 budget for the day (and then some), so you do need to be careful about the quantities of seeds and nuts you consume, even if they're in their natural state.

Seeds and nuts are not a critical part of our diet and should be consumed sparingly (especially seeds). If you treat seeds as a garnish and nuts as an occasional treat then you won't go wrong. The chart below sets out the fat content of the more popular seeds and nuts. As always, if your favourite isn't there, then look it up on my free foods database at davidgillespie.org.

Fat breakdown of raw nuts and seeds

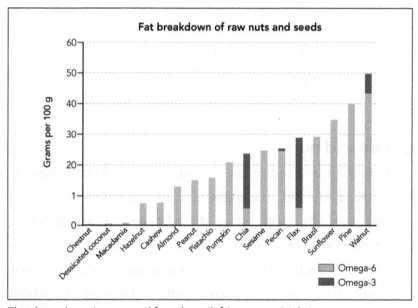

The chart above is arranged from best (left) to worst (right).

Anything to the right of pistachio nuts (except flaxseed, which contains omega-3 rather than omega-6) should be avoided if you're eating serious quantities.

One hundred grams of nuts or seeds – more than 2 cups of sunflower seeds and about 70 cashew nuts – is an awful lot to scoff in a sitting. But if you're tempted to eat that many, it's best to stick to macadamias or you'll be blowing your daily polyunsaturated-fat budget in one fell swoop.

> **If all you're doing is sprinkling some seeds
> over your porridge or using them in a recipe,
> then their fat content isn't a worry.**

Assembled foods and shortcuts

After you've separated out the real food and the fake food, you'll find you have a bunch of foods that aren't in either category. I could have made a simple (and simplistic) rule and said if it's in a packet, jar or box and has a list of ingredients, it's not real food and it should go. But out here in the real world, there are things that are just plain useful that it would be good to be able to buy pre-assembled.

For example, I like hot chips. As you're about to discover, I can't buy them from 99 per cent of takeaway joints because they're fried in seed oils. Yes, I could cut up potatoes, boil them and then double-fry them in animal fat, but who's got the time for that every time they want chips? (Although if you do, there's a recipe for doing just that in Chapter 10.) So I use supermarket-bought frozen chips (intended for oven-frying). This is a processed food and wouldn't be allowed in an absolute rule against fake food. But knowledge is power, and as long as we're careful about exactly what we buy, we can navigate our way through some savings in time and effort with some fake foods. These will be foods that are largely processed but that may be acceptable depending on which ingredients the manufacturer has chosen to use. The rest of this section is devoted to helping you figure out what do to about them.

The foods in this section are assembled and processed foods. They come in boxes and packets but, with a bit of label reading (for which I'm about to give you some shortcuts), you can quickly sort the good brands from the bad. Throughout these sections I'll apply two sets of rules: one for sugar content and one for seed-oil content. If the product fails either test you should avoid it, but you may still be able to buy something similar that doesn't fail the tests. Because you'll almost certainly be replacing all of these foods with something similar, I've also included tips on what to look for and what your options will be.

The sugar and fat rules

To see how these rules work, let's examine this nice box of Arnott's Chicken Crimpy Shapes cracker biscuits.

FLAVOURED BISCUITS

INGREDIENTS	NUTRITION INFORMATION		
Wheat Flour, Vegetable Oil, Sugar, Salt, Malt Extract (From Barley), Raising Agents (E500, E341), Flavour Enhancers (E621, E635, Chicken, Onion Powder, Yeast Extract, Antioxidants (E306 From Soy, E304), Natural Flavour, Emulsifier (E322 From Soy). **MAY CONTAIN TRACES OF EGG, MILK, NUT AND SESAME.**	SERVINGS PER PACKAGE: 7	SERVING SIZE: 25g	
	QUANTITY PER SERVING	%DAILY INTAKE* PER SERVING	QUANTITY PER 100g
	ENERGY 490kJ	5.6%	1960kJ
	PROTEIN 1.9g	3.9%	7.8g
	FAT – total 4.9g	7.0%	19.7g
	– saturated 1.0g	4.1%	4.0g
	CARBOHYDRATE 15.8g	5.1%	63.3g
	– sugars 1.8g	2.0%	7.1g
	SODIUM 240mg	10.4%	958mg
	* PERCENTAGE DAILY INTAKES ARE BASED ON AN AVERAGE ADULT DIET OF 8700 KJ. YOUR DAILY INTAKES MAY BE HIGHER OR LOWER DEPENDING ON YOUR ENERGY NEEDS. **ALL VALUES CONSIDERED AVERAGES UNLESS OTHERWISE INDICATED.**		

THE SUGAR RULES

Looking at the nutrition information on the Arnott's Chicken Crimpy Shapes cracker biscuits box, let's ask a couple of questions.

Q1 Is there a bad sweetener sugar in the ingredients list (see the 'Sweetener cheat sheet' above)? (This is rule 1.)

A Yes, there is – sugar.

Q2 If there is, then is the total sugar more than 3 grams per 100 grams? (This is rule 2.)

A Yes, it is – it's 7.1 grams per 100 grams.

Since the answer to both of these questions is yes, the product fails the sugar rules and must be thrown out. There are, however, two exceptions to the sugar rule – dairy products and drinks.

Dairy products

These contain lactose and it should be less than 5 grams per 100 grams. The only trouble is that 5 grams will be lumped in with

NUTRITIONAL INFORMATION		
Servings per package: 3		
Serving size: 150 g		
	Quantity per Serving	Quantity per 100 g
Energy	608 kJ	405 kJ
Protein	4.2 g	2.8 g
Fat, total	7.4 g	4.9 g
– saturated	4.5 g	3.0 g
Carbohydrate, total	18.6 g	12.4 g
– sugars	18.6 g	12.4 g
Sodium	90 mg	60 mg
Calcium	300 mh (38%)*	200 mg
* Percentage of recommended dietary intake		
Ingredients: Whole milk, concentrated skim milk, sugar, strawberries (9%), gelatine, culture, thickener (1442).		

any added sugar on the label. This means that rule 2 is modified to lift the acceptable limit to 8 grams per 100 grams for dairy products (such as yoghurt and ice-cream).

The label above is for a tub of strawberry yoghurt. It has 12.4 grams of sugar per 100 grams, but the first 5 grams of that will be perfectly acceptable lactose. So its added sugar content is 12.4 – 5 = 7.4 grams. Since that is still above our 3-gram limit, this would be going in the bin.

Drinks

When we drink, we generally consume much more than 100 grams (100 millilitres) of drink – a can of soft drink is almost 400 grams worth, for example – so we can't apply the same generous allowance.

For drinks rule 2 is dropped to 0 grams per 100 grams. This means that pretty much the only acceptable non-alcoholic drinks become milk (remember, it's a dairy product, so it gets a 5 grams per 100 grams head start) and water. If that sounds boring, I guess you aren't really thirsty.

Food manufacturers aren't required to identify the exact fats they're using in a product, but they are required to tell us the total fat in grams per 100 grams and the saturated fat in grams per 100 grams. Using those two numbers and the rules below, the trained seed-oil detective can have a good guess as to the type of fat being used based on the amount of saturated fat in the product.

THE SEED-OIL RULE

You'll be chucking them out because of the sugar content, but just for consistency, once again let's use the Chicken Crimpy Shapes label and ask this question.

Q1   Is there a bad oil in the ingredients list (see the 'Fats and oils cheat sheet' above)?

A   Yes, there is – vegetable oil (You'll see this a lot rather than a specific oil name. The trouble is that palm oils and coconut oils are vegetable oils as well, so this doesn't tell you much about the actual fat used – it could be a seed oil or it could be a good oil.)

Now divide the saturated fat per 100 grams (4.0 grams) by the total fat per 100 grams (19.7 grams) and then multiply by 100 to obtain the percentage of the product that's saturated fat.

$$4.0/19.7 = 0.203$$

$$0.203 \times 100 = 20.3\%$$

Now see where that percentage lands on the following graph.

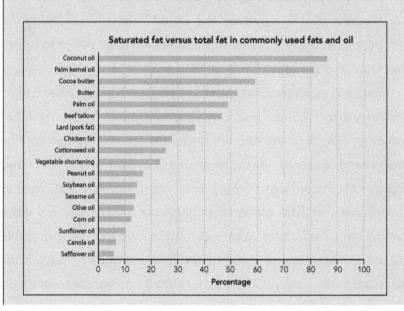

Saturated fat versus total fat in commonly used fats and oil

That reveals that the fat in the product is probably vegetable shortening, a blend of cottonseed oil and soybean oil. Since both of those are seed oils that are very high in the dangerous polyunsaturated fats, we know we're best off throwing the product out.

As a general rule, the lower the percentage you get, the more likely you should avoid the product. The only real exception to that is products that use olive oil (because of its high monounsaturated-fat content) and believe me, if they're using that, they'll make sure you know it (because it's an expensive ingredient).

Butter

Since the invention of cows (of the domestic variety), butter has been the spread of choice whenever mankind encountered bread. It's a cheap cooking and eating fat that can be made by anybody prepared to invest elbow grease. To people alive before the First World War, the thought of using anything else would be absurd. Dripping (fat left over from cooking meat) was also occasionally added to bread, but more as a sandwich filling or topping than as a spread.

Butter is much more spreadable if you leave it out of the fridge, but in warmer climes that can be problematic. The only other solution is to fork out the big bucks for spreadable butter. The only brand of spreadable butter available in Australia is Mainland Buttersoft. It contains nothing but cream and salt and, in that respect, is just like butter. Straight from the fridge, it's more spreadable than butter (although only about half as spreadable as margarine) because some of the harder saturated fatty acids have been removed (reducing its saturated-fat content from about

54 per cent to about 52 per cent). It's nutritionally equivalent to butter and there's no downside to using it (other than the price).

Don't fall for labelling that says 'dairy blend'. It's not butter (no matter how many times it says 'made with real butter' or uses the word 'buttery' on the front of the pack). These franken-products are made by mixing margarine and butter together to make the butter more spreadable straight from the fridge. The major blends available in Australia are Devondale Dairy Soft, Western Star spreads (but not their butter) and the supermarket generic 'dairy blends'. If in doubt, check the ingredient list. If it says anything other than cream, water and salt, it's not butter.

WHAT IS BUTTER (AND GHEE)?

Butter is made by boiling milk to separate the cream, then churning the cream until the fat separates from the buttermilk (the runny bit). If you plan to keep it for a while then it might be a good idea to add a bit of salt as a preservative. You can do it yourself right now. No special equipment is required (although I recommend buying cream as a starting point to cut yourself a little slack).

To make ghee, just heat the butter. It will 'split', meaning the fat solids will separate from any remaining milk proteins. Ghee has a much higher smoke point than butter (see below for info on smoke points and what they mean) so (unlike butter) can be used in the deep-fryer.

You may have some olive-oil margarine in your fridge and you might be thinking that since olive oil is on the good list you can keep it. If those margarines were actually made from olive oil that would be true, but because its melting point is −40°C, olive oil can't be made into a solid margarine. So, no matter how many pictures of olives appear on the front of that olive-oil spread, it's a blend of olive oil and seed oils – and usually only about one-third of the oil used is from olives. Chuck it out.

Breads

Most bread recipes use fat. In the olden days (before the Second World War), that fat was usually some form of animal fat (often lard). Now almost all commercially produced bread you're likely to encounter uses some added sugar as well as a seed oil (usually canola, but sometimes soybean or sunflower). The good news is that it generally won't be much of either, so if you can't come at making your own, there are some low-seed-oil alternatives. Just remember, it all counts, so be careful how much of a seed-oil-loaded bread you consume.

BEST SUPERMARKET WHITES (IF YOU MUST PURCHASE A SUPERMARKET WHITE)

- Coles Smart Buy White (0.8 gram of polyunsaturated fat and 1.8 grams of sugar per 100 grams – 3 slices)
- Tip Top The One, Tip Top Sunblest White or Tip Top UP White plus 25 per cent wholegrain (about the same polyunsaturated-fat content, slightly more sugar but still under 3 grams per 100 grams)
- Woolworths White (0.9 gram polyunsaturated fat but a little too much sugar – 3.2 grams per 100 grams)

The best non-white bread is Bürgen Rye, but be aware that it contains a little under twice the amount of polyunsaturated fat (1.4 grams per 100 grams – two and a bit slices). If the only bread you eat is a couple of slices of Bürgen Rye toast in the morning, then that won't matter much. But if that bread is a big part of your daily diet, then you will need to be careful – five slices will blow your entire daily budget for polyunsaturated fats.

Sourdough is usually a good choice because traditional recipes call for neither sugar nor fat. Unfortunately, that doesn't stop some supermarket brands adding a dash of canola oil, so check the label before you toss it in the trolley.

Bakers are also big fans of vegetable oil. A loaf of bread uses $0.04 worth of canola oil whereas the same amount of olive oil would cost $0.20. So I suspect their preference is mostly a cost thing because there would be nothing wrong (even on current standard health advice) with using olive oil. We've found, however, that you can ask your baker to use olive oil instead and they're prepared to do it (as long as you order ahead). Better still, they don't even charge you the extra $0.16!

Wraps

There are some good oil- and sugar-free choices with wraps, so an effective way to circumvent the whole bread question is to go for the flattened variety. Mountain Bread brand doesn't use added sugar or oil in any of its range. Mission and Tip Top both add vegetable oil and sugar, and even though the Mission Lite Wrap has the lowest polyunsaturated-fat content of any wrap, it's too high in sugar (5 grams per 100 grams). For gluten-free options, choose wraps made from rice or corn flour, but check the label for added sugar and avoid products with more than 3 grams per 100 grams.

Flour

Even if a manufacturer adds no oils to their bread or wrap, these products will still contain polyunsaturated fat. Grains are seeds and flour is made from grains. But not all grains are equal when it comes to fat content. The graph below shows polyunsaturated-fat content per 100 grams (about the amount in two to three slices of bread) for the common flours. Clearly, anything made with soy flour or almond should be avoided. A couple of slices of bread made with that stuff will take out your daily polyunsaturated fat budget for two whole days before you even look at what else you

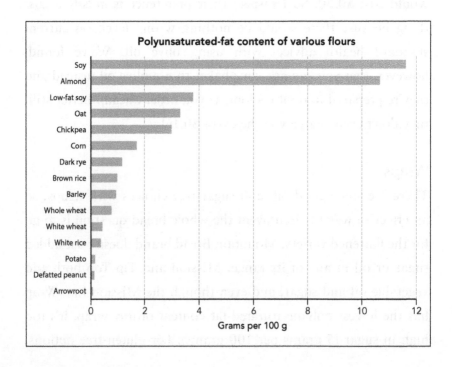

eat or what you spread on the bread. Reduced-fat soy is better, but even then its polyunsaturated-fat content is twice as high as the next worse, corn flour. Potato and rice flour are great choices for the gluten-intolerant, and wheat flour is a good choice for the rest of us.

If you're inclined to do a bit of DIY (see next section), keep this graph handy when choosing flours.

DIY

Of course doing (making) it yourself is the best way to ensure you know exactly what's in your bread ... if you do that, you'll know for certain that it contains neither added seed oil nor added sugar, and you'll probably halve your daily consumption of both (from bread).

Making bread is nowhere near as hard as television chefs make it look. Give it a go (see the recipes in Chapter Ten). By the way, we've noticed that since Lizzie started making all our own bread, everyone in the house tends to eat less of it. And no, it's not because it tastes bad (quite the opposite), it's because it's much less available. Bread becomes a freshly baked, gorgeous-smelling treat rather than something you have just because it's there.

Spreads (other than butter)

Now you've got the bread sorted out, you might want to splash out on something to put on it (other than butter). The sugar content will have meant you've already chucked out the honey, jam and Nutella, but you might still have a jar of peanut butter (or other nut butter) and some Vegemite on hand. Vegemite contains no added oils and very little sugar, so you can hang on to that. Peanut butter is a trickier proposition. Peanuts are relatively high in polyunsaturated fats (at 14.9 grams per 100 grams) and so, therefore, is anything made from them. To make it worse, sugar is also often added to peanut butter.

The best peanut butter (on the fat front) is Kraft Light, and the option with the lowest sugar content is Sanitarium No Added Sugar or Salt. To get the best of both worlds, it's best to go for Sanitarium No Added Sugar or Salt or the Coles brand peanut butter (not Coles Smart Buy, which doesn't display its polyunsaturated-fat content, but the standard Coles brand). If you have a standard serving (25 grams or 1 tablespoon or two pieces of toast's worth) of either of these, you'll be notching up about 1.2 grams of omega-6 polyunsaturated fat. Oddly, that's quite a bit less than in a peanut itself (which has 4 grams of omega-6 in the same-sized serve).

If you're asking yourself (as I did) why there's so much less polyunsaturated fat in most of the commercial brands, it's because they don't start from raw peanuts. Rather, commercial peanut butter is made from peanut flour that's been partially de-fatted. This lowers the total fat content of the end product and increases the protein, both of which are good if you're selling a high-fat product to a fat-wary consumer. For once, the public paranoia about fat works in favour of those of us avoiding polyunsaturated fats as well. We receive a reasonable selection of low-polyunsaturated-fat peanut butters in the supermarket, leaving us with only the added sugar to worry about.

You can, of course, make your own peanut butter. All you need is some form of blender or food processor (or a desire for a workout), peanuts and a pinch of salt. But I really wouldn't bother if I were you. In this instance the commercial varieties made with low-fat peanut powder are a better option from an omega-6 perspective.

If other nut butters take your fancy, flip back to the 'Fat breakdown of raw nuts' chart on page 138 to see their relative goodness or badness. Walnut butter, for example, would be a very bad choice, but if you're feeling wealthy, you can do a lot better by having your nut butter made from macadamias. Macadamia nut spread has almost no polyunsaturated fats and no more sugar than whole macadamia nuts (4.5 grams per 100 grams).

You could, of course, raid Mother Nature's supermarket instead and break out the avocados. There's nothing nicer than avocado mashed into a piece of homemade hot buttered sourdough toast seasoned with a little salt and pepper (or even lemon juice). Avocado has almost no sugar, but a medium-sized (240-gram) avocado will have about 4.3 grams of polyunsaturated fat, so it's a good idea to keep the serving to about a quarter of a fruit (providing about 1 gram of polyunsaturated fat) in any one sitting.

Condiments

Having applied the sugar rules will mean you'll have given most condiments the flick, since sugar is the primary ingredient in just about every 'savoury' sauce (see below). Most condiments are the dietary equivalent of adding a couple (or more) teaspoons of sugar to every serving of everything you eat. Sauce is one of the sneaky sources (get it?) of added sugar that almost nobody takes into account when they tell me they don't eat much sugar.

Sauce	Sugar content
Barbecue	48–55%
Hoisin	50%
Steak	45%
Sweet chilli	43–49%
Chocolate	40%
Brown (for example, HP)	26%
Ketchup	25%
Worcestershire	15–36%
Tomato	21–36%
Low-fat mayonnaise	21%
Apple	15%
Tartare	6–10%
Fish	6%
Laksa	5%
Pesto	2–5%
Salad dressings	0–6%
Taco	1.5%
Soy	1%
Whole-egg mayonnaise	<1%
Tabasco	0

Whole-egg mayonnaise, some pestos and salad dressings might have survived the sugar rules, but unfortunately, with very few exceptions, they won't get past the seed-oil rule.

Mayonnaise

No one's sure who came up with the first recipe for mayonnaise. The Spanish reckon it came from Mahon in Spain and was nicked by the French in 1756. The French reckon they had it for ages before that. They say it was named after the Duke of Mayenne when he took the time to finish his chicken and mayo sanger before the Battle of Arques in 1589.

But wherever it came from, there's general agreement on the recipe. You grab an egg yolk and whisk in olive oil. It's a cool bit of chemistry for two such simple ingredients. The oil and the water in the yolk create an emulsion that's stabilised by the proteins and lecithin in the yolk. If you want to get all fancy, you can drop in a bit of mustard or lemon juice to give it a sharper tang.

And that's all there is to one of the yummiest and most widespread condiments in the world today. Except, apparently, if you're a food conglomerate trying to make a fat-free mayo. Given that 80 per cent of the product is fat (olive oil) this presents a wee problem. Don't worry, though, there's a solution – pack it with sugar instead. For example, Praise Creamy Mayonnaise is 97 per cent fat-free. And while the label claims this is 'mayonnaise', the ingredients list doesn't look like anything the Duke of Mayenne is likely to have used. There's neither egg nor olive oil involved in its construction. Indeed, the primary ingredient (besides water) is sugar. Here's the full ingredients list (in descending order of use in the product).

PRAISE CREAMY 97% FAT-FREE MAYONNAISE INGREDIENTS

Water (about 70%)	Lemon juice
Sugar (26.8%)	Sunflower oil (0.8%)
Vinegar	Spices
Thickener (1442)	Colour (171, lutein)
Salt	Food acid (citric)
Vegetable gums (415, 460, 466)	Flavour

Based on the volumes of each ingredient used, this 'mayonnaise' is really just a sugar-water emulsion flavoured with a bit of salt, vinegar and sunflower oil (0.8 per cent of the total volume – there's more lemon juice than oil in this baby). Low-fat mayonnaise in general contains huge amounts of sugar (often well over 20 per cent), so you'll have binned that already. Whole-egg mayonnaise, on the other hand, is very low in sugar – most brands are less than 2 per cent sugar and quite a few are zero. The only one you need watch out for is Praise's reduced-fat whole-egg mayo, which is 13 per cent sugar. Non-egg-based mayos, marketed as 'traditional mayonnaise', have around 8.5 per cent sugar in the full-fat versions and up to 21 per cent sugar in the reduced-fat versions, so avoid them at all costs.

But if you're a mayo fan, you still need to tread carefully. Most of the big-brand mayos are made from sunflower oil, one of the nastiest seed oils. We haven't been able to find a commercial mayonnaise made from olive oil at anything approaching a reasonable price. This is a bit of a problem in our house, because the twins in particular love the stuff on just about everything. Thankfully, we have an eldest child who really doesn't seem to mind powering up the food processor when more is needed. He gets a lot of adulation from his little sisters for something that takes him approximately five seconds, so I reckon he thinks that's a fair deal. The recipe is in Chapter 10.

Unfortunately, traditional mayo is used as the basis for commercial coleslaw, so you can expect a big serve of sugar and seed oil if you buy pre-made coleslaw from the supermarket. You can, of course, make it yourself and it's very quick and easy (the recipe is in *Toxic Oil*), but another alternative is to buy precut coleslaw vegetables (from the fruit and veg section of the supermarket) and add your own homemade mayo. I defy you or your sugar- and seed-oil-munching friends to detect the difference between the commercial product and your homemade coleslaw, but it's almost – except for the carrot and cabbage – sugar-free and, if you've made your own mayo or shopped in the premium aisle, it's also seed-oil-free.

Pestos

Commercial pestos and dips are a seed-oil minefield. Just as with mayo, the fat of choice for almost all manufacturers is now sunflower or canola oil. And because of the nature of the product, these oils are usually the primary ingredient. As far as I know, the only exceptions to that rule are Black Swan Corn Relish and Saclà Black Olive Paté.

Fortunately, most basic sauces and pestos are commercial copies of recipes that have been handmade using olive oil for generations. I've tested (in the sense that Lizzie made them and I ate them) a large number of these traditional recipes, and collected the best and the easiest to make in *Toxic Oil*.

Salad dressings

You're going to need to get used to eating salads au naturel or with homemade dressings. Some brands have absolutely no fat and therefore no polyunsaturated fat, but every standard serving (20 grams or 1.25 tablespoons) will deliver a big lump of sugar (at least half and usually a whole teaspoon's worth). The low-sugar options mean a huge serve of polyunsaturated fat instead. All the commercial dressings that contain fat are based on sunflower, rice bran, canola or soybean oil, and pretty much all the polyunsaturated-fat numbers are ugly. If you can't get through the day without salad dressing, your best choice is probably the Praise Italian 100% Fat Free. It will still give you half a teaspoon of sugar in a single serve, but if you only have one serve and that's all the sugar you're consuming that day, it's not going to kill you. Once again, making your own is the best option. If you want some recipes, I provided a selection in *Toxic Oil*.

Non-dairy milk

Cow's milk contains sugar. It's lactose and it's metabolised to glucose by humans, so it's not a concern to us fructose-avoiders. But when imitation milks are manufactured from soy, rice or almonds, the makers invariably use cane sugar (sucrose) as the sugar. This means they're almost all unacceptably high in fructose. There are, however, three fructose-free alternatives: Pureharvest, which uses rice malt syrup (essentially glucose); Vitasoy's Protein Enriched Rice Milk, which isn't sweetened at all; and Bonsoy Soy Milk, which is sweetened with tapioca syrup (also glucose). The bad news is that none of these products has anything approaching a safe level of polyunsaturated fat.

The chart below sets out most of the brands of milk alternative on sale in Australia today in ascending order of polyunsaturated-fat content from left to right. Almost all soy-, rice- and almond-based 'milks' are made with either sunflower or canola oil (or sometimes both). Even those that don't have added oil still contain significant quantities of polyunsaturated fat from the base ingredient (if it's soybeans or almonds). The best choice is probably the Vitasoy Oatmilk. It has neither added sugar nor added oil.

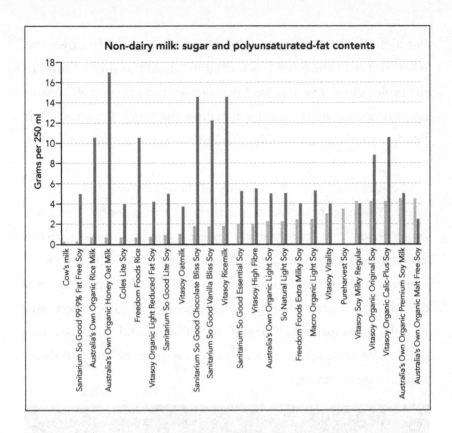

Non-dairy milk: sugar and polyunsaturated-fat contents

If you're avoiding cow's milk because of lactose intolerance, one of the enzyme-treated milks (such as Pauls Zymil) is the way to go. It's ordinary cow's milk treated with the lactase enzyme that lactose-intolerant people are missing, which means the lactose has been disassembled into its component galactose and glucose, and should present no problems for people with lactose in tolerance.

Yoghurt

Yoghurt is quite tart in its natural state. That might come as a bit of a surprise to many Australians, because the vast majority of what we're sold as 'yoghurt' has more in common with ice-cream than Greek yoghurt. Plain yoghurt does contain sugar, but as in milk, it's lactose (which doesn't contain fructose). So when you read the label you'll need to adjust the sugar figure. In the table below, I've assumed that lactose accounts for 4.7 grams per 100 grams of the sugars listed on the label. It varies a fair bit, but that's a reasonable average for the sake of comparing brands.

Besides the diet yoghurts, none of the yoghurts listed will taste sweet. You might not like to eat them by the spoonful, but you'd be surprised how scrumptious they get if you mix in some berries and maybe a bit of vanilla or dextrose or both. Plain yoghurt is a great thing to have in the fridge even if you don't plan to eat it straight. It's a great base for salad dressings, a good alternative to milk in recipes (see Chapter 10 for why) and is terrific as a topping for fruit salad, especially if you toast some coconut flakes and mix them through.

Label	Sugar content (%)	Adjusted sugar content (%)
Jalna BioDynamic Organic Whole Milk	4.1	0
Chobani Non-Fat Plain	4.1	0
Chobani Low-Fat Plain	4.1	0
Nestlé Soleil Diet Mixed Berry	4.1	0
Nestlé Soleil Diet Passionfruit	4.1	0
Nestlé Soleil Diet Fruit Salad	4.2	0
Nestlé Soleil Diet Vanilla	4.4	0
Nestlé Soleil Diet Black Cherry	4.5	0
Nestlé Soleil Diet Strawberry	4.5	0
Nestlé Soleil Diet Peach & Mango	4.6	0
Yoplait Formé Sticky Date	4.6	0
Yoplait Formé Strawberry	4.6	0
Yoplait Formé French Vanilla	4.7	0

Label	Sugar content (%)	Adjusted sugar content (%)
Tamar Valley Greek Style No Added Sugar Strawberry	4.8	0.1
Jalna Greek Natural	4.8	0.1
Macro Wholefoods Market Organic Greek Style	4.9	0.2
Yoplait Formé Raspberry	4.9	0.2
Yoplait Formé Peach Mango	5.0	0.3
Yoplait Formé Tropical	5.0	0.3
Tamar Valley Greek Style No Added Sugar Mixed Berry	5.0	0.3
Yoplait Formé Field Berries	5.1	0.4
Yoplait Formé Passionfruit	5.1	0.4
Jalna Leben European Style	5.2	0.5
Black Swan Greek Style Naturally Sweet	5.4	0.7
Jalna Fat Free Natural	5.5	0.8
Brooklea Lite Natural	5.5	0.8
Five:am Natural No Added Sugar	5.6	0.9
Jalna a2 Low Fat Natural	5.6	0.9
Woolworths Select Greek Style	5.8	1.1
Black Swan Greek Style Naturally Sweet No Fat	5.9	1.2
Gippsland Dairy Organic Natural	6.1	1.4
Just Organic Natural	6.3	1.6
Liddells Lactose Free Plain	6.4	1.7
Black Swan Greek Style Vanilla Bean	6.5	1.8
Farmers Union European Style Natural	6.5	1.8
Pauls All Natural 99.8% Fat Free	6.5	1.8
Coles Natural Set	6.6	1.9
Jalna Greek Low Fat Natural	6.7	2.0
Jalna Premium Creamy Natural	6.7	2.0
Tamar Valley Greek Style No Added Sugar Raspberry	6.8	2.1
Lyttos Lite Greek Style Natural	7.0	2.3
Farmers Union Greek Style Natural	7.2	2.5
Tamar Valley Greek Style No Added Sugar Mango	7.4	2.7

Breakfast cereals

The only cereals that contain even remotely acceptable levels of sugar are variations on (unflavoured) oats and wheat biscuits (provided, of course, you don't add sugar or honey yourself). There's quite a good selection of puffed grains available in the health-food sections of both major supermarkets. You can find no-sugar, no-oil versions of rice bubbles, puffed Kamut and even puffed corn. But these things are pricey, and if your kids eat anything like the way ours do, you'll probably be looking for a cheaper option. The cheapest cereal with the lowest sugar content (and no seed oils) we've discovered is the Coles generic brand wheat biscuits. Uncle Tobys Vita Brits and Oatbrits are also good if you prefer something with a brand. Our kids will eat them when no one can be bothered cooking an egg or a sausage or mashing up an avocado on toast, but they're hardly choice number one. Frankly, you get over having cereal for breakfast once you've been eating real food for a while.

Potato-based products

Obviously potatoes are real food. And they can be cooked loads of different ways, which makes them an interesting addition to any meal or even a meal on their own. I have, of course, included recipes for some of our favourite preparation methods in Chapter 10. But here I'll give you a guide to the shortcuts in the world of potatoes. This is especially important if you're partial (as I am) to having your potatoes fried.

Chips

Like, I suspect, most adult Australians, before deciding to eat real food I'd never deep-fried anything. Anti-fat political correctness now ensures that most of us are terrified of fat and the closest we'll come to a home-cooked chip is to 'oven-fry' a bag of frozen chips. But like most things, it's not as hard to do it yourself as it might seem. All you need are potatoes, a pot and some animal fat. We use Supafry (a blend of animal fats), which you can get in most supermarkets (in the butter section). If you'd prefer to use a plant-based fat, then either refined (light or mild) olive oil or coconut oil is fine too.

To make your own, chop some potatoes into chips (which you can do with a device for such things or a plain old knife), boil them until cooked, then drain and cool them. Once they're cold, pre-fry the chips at around 160°C, then refry them at 190–200°C. It's a bit time-consuming, but when the kids and I really want proper chips, I do it. You'll find the recipe in Chapter 10.

If you want to make life easier, you can buy frozen chips. They're marketed as 'oven-fry chips' but that's just 'political correctness'. They're exactly the same as the chips that every fast-food joint is tossing into their boiling seed oil. They're not seed-oil-free, as I'll explain in a moment, but they're acceptable if you fry them in animal fat or olive oil.

Frozen chips are pieces of potato that have been pre-fried in seed (usually canola) oil. Obviously this isn't ideal for us real-food eaters, but because most of the fat is absorbed in the second frying, doing that final fry in animal fat means we significantly reduce the amount of polyunsaturated fat we eat (compared to getting the same thing from a shop or restaurant).

The amount of polyunsaturated fat in the chip is influenced by the oil used and the thickness of the chip (thinner chips means more fat per 100 grams of potato), so the amount varies quite a bit between brands. To save you some time, I've had a look through the supermarket for you. The best I could find was McCain Healthy Choice Straight Cut (0.7 gram per 100 grams). But other good choices include McCain Healthy Choice Chunky Cut (0.8 gram), Birds Eye Curly Fries (0.8 gram), McCain Superfries Mum or Straight Cut (0.9 gram), Birds Eye or Coles Steakhouse (1 gram) and McCain Original Crunchy, Hot Bandito Wedges and Original Wedges (all 1 gram).

Deep-frying the McCain Healthy Choice Straight Cut chips in animal fat will probably add about half a gram of polyunsaturated fat to the total (which brings it to 1.2 grams). While that total ends up being around half a gram of polyunsaturated fat more than if you went to the trouble of making the chips yourself, it's still an awfully long way short of the 5.3 grams you'd get from 100 grams of McDonald's fries (a 'medium' fries).

Hash browns and other assorted frozen-potato products

Most oven-fry potato products are prepared the same way. Unfortunately, almost all the other varieties of hash browns and gems end up with more than twice as much polyunsaturated fat as chips.

This means that if you eat just four frozen hash browns (about 300 grams) you'll have exceeded your daily 6 grams polyunsaturated fat limit. (And if you get them at McDonald's, just two hash browns will do it.) If it's not a complete fry-up for you without hash browns from a packet, then choose McCain Hash Browns (2.4 grams of polyunsaturated fat per 100 grams), just have one and, as much as possible, stay away from polyunsaturated fats for the rest of the day. Of course, you could just make your own. I've provided a simple hash brown recipe in *Toxic Oil*. If potato gems are what you'd prefer, the best choice is Birds Eye Golden Crunch Potato Gems (2.1 grams per 100 grams). These are the numbers if you oven-fry them. If you deep-fry them you can add at least another 0.5 gram polyunsaturated fat per 100 grams.

Potato crisps and corn chips

Crisps are a reasonable treat to have around, especially when you're asking kids (in particular) to go without sugar. And there's not a lot wrong with them on the real food front, as long as you're careful which ones you choose. Australian plain (just salted) crisps are usually fried in either sunflower or palm oil. But there's a twist. The oil being used isn't the ordinary sunflower oil, it's the oil from a type of sunflower bred to produce seed oils extremely low in polyunsaturated fats, called high-oleic sunflower oil (which is why this particular type of sunflower oil is on the good list on page 118).

There's a large variation in the total fat content of plain salted crisps. Some have about the same amount of total fat as hot chips (around 20 grams per 100 grams), while others have almost double that. Because the total fat varies a lot, so does the amount of polyunsaturated fat, regardless of which oil was used to cook the chips.

When you start browsing the chippie aisle, you'll discover that Grain Waves appear a reasonable option on the basis of fat content, but they also contain 5.1 grams of sugar per 100 grams so should be avoided. The Red Rock Deli Sea Salt potato chips come out as the best choice (1.5 grams of polyunsaturated fat per 100 grams) but most brands are less than double that. The only ones you need avoid are Macro Organic Gluten Free Chips (9.4 grams per 100 grams) and the Red Rock Deli Corn Chips (5 grams per 100 grams). Bear in mind that 100 grams of chips is quite a lot. The lunch-box-size packs of potato chips that come in big boxes of twenty (or so) weigh only 19 grams each (so they can claim to be only 100 calories) and probably represent a reasonable child-sized serve. Even if an adult ate two of those in a sitting, they'd consume just half a gram (Red Rock) to 1 gram (most others) of polyunsaturated fat.

Unfortunately, this advice really only relates to unflavoured (plain, salted) chips. Once you venture into flavoured varieties, the oils once again veer into the usual concoction of seed oils, and many of them also have considerable amounts of sugar. If salt and vinegar or sour cream and chives are more your thing, you'll need to use the sweetener and seed-oil rules above to figure out if you can have them.

Chicken-based products

Real-food eaters cannot live on chips alone, so I've included some batter and crumbing recipes at the end of the book and some more in *Toxic Oil*. Just buy chicken (or fish) fillets and crumb or batter them before dropping them in boiling animal fat – yum! If you have neither the time nor the inclination to get up to your elbows in batter or crumbing mix (it can be messy and time-consuming), there are some 'oven-fry' options in the freezer section of the supermarket. I don't really recommend any of them – even those lowest in polyunsaturated fat will put a fair old dent in your 6 grams per day allowance (with just six nuggets). But if you must, select items from the top of the list below, in order to minimise the impact.

Chicken (-based) product	Grams of polyunsaturated fat per 100 g
Raw chicken breast*	0.7
Ingham Crumbed Breast Fillets	3.3
Steggles Chicken Breast Fingers	3.5
Steggles Chicken Breast Chunks	4.1
Steggles Chicken Fingers and Chicken Crackles	4.5
Steggles Chicken Strips Southern Style	4.6
Steggles Chicken Strips Peri Peri	4.7

Chicken (-based) product	Grams of polyunsaturated fat per 100 g
Steggles Chicken Fingers Salt & Vinegar	5.5
Ingham Chicken Breast Schnitzel	5.5
McDonald's Chicken McNuggets (cooked)**	5.5
Steggles Chicken Nuggets Dino Snacks and Fairy Snacks	5.6
Ingham Chickadee Chicken Tenders	5.8
Steggles Chicken Little Tenders	7.1
Ingham Chickadee Chicken Chips	7.3
Steggles Chicken Nuggets Premium	7.4
Ingham Chickadee Chicken & Cheese Schnitzel	7.5
Ingham Chicken Burgers	7.7
Steggles Chicken Nuggets Value	8.6

* I've included a raw chicken breast as a comparison, just so you know how much to allow for the chicken itself.

** I've also included McDonald's Chicken McNuggets as a comparison. One hundred grams (about six) of these is likely to contain around 5.5 grams of polyunsaturated fat. If you purchased some chicken breast meat and crumbed or battered some 'nuggets', then deep-fried them in animal fat, the end result would contain 1.2–1.5 grams of polyunsaturated fat. You'd be consuming around 4 grams less polyunsaturated fat than if you bought nuggets from Macca's, and 2.5–8 grams less than if you started from a box of frozen chicken(ish) product and deep-fried them in animal fat. You'd also have the advantage of knowing that your nugget was all breast chicken.

Fish-based products

Fish in general contains more polyunsaturated fat than other types of meat we might encounter, so when comparing fish-based assembled food, we should always have an eye to what the unadulterated meat contains. That's why I've included examples of raw fish meat (marked with *) in the table below.

Once again, if your favourite isn't on the list, take a look at the free food database at davidgillespie.org.

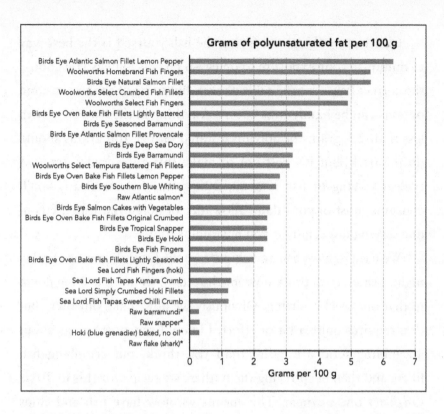

Grams of polyunsaturated fat per 100 g

	Grams per 100 g
Birds Eye Atlantic Salmon Fillet Lemon Pepper	
Woolworths Homebrand Fish Fingers	
Birds Eye Natural Salmon Fillet	
Woolworths Select Crumbed Fish Fillets	
Woolworths Select Fish Fingers	
Birds Eye Oven Bake Fish Fillets Lightly Battered	
Birds Eye Seasoned Barramundi	
Birds Eye Atlantic Salmon Fillet Provencale	
Birds Eye Deep Sea Dory	
Birds Eye Barramundi	
Woolworths Select Tempura Battered Fish Fillets	
Birds Eye Oven Bake Fish Fillets Lemon Pepper	
Birds Eye Southern Blue Whiting	
Raw Atlantic salmon*	
Birds Eye Salmon Cakes with Vegetables	
Birds Eye Oven Bake Fish Fillets Original Crumbed	
Birds Eye Tropical Snapper	
Birds Eye Hoki	
Birds Eye Fish Fingers	
Birds Eye Oven Bake Fish Fillets Lightly Seasoned	
Sea Lord Fish Fingers (hoki)	
Sea Lord Fish Tapas Kumara Crumb	
Sea Lord Simply Crumbed Hoki Fillets	
Sea Lord Fish Tapas Sweet Chilli Crumb	
Raw barramundi*	
Raw snapper*	
Hoki (blue grenadier) baked, no oil*	
Raw flake (shark)*	

Somewhat surprisingly (given we're constantly told to eat more fish), Atlantic salmon is the only raw fish that contains significant quantities of polyunsaturated fat. Because they really don't need insulation, tropical fish (the ones we're most likely to encounter in Australia) like barramundi and hoki have almost no fat to speak of. Careful label-reading will reveal most 'fish' products used in frozen food are actually hoki (blue grenadier, caught in New Zealand, Chile and Argentina, then exported to China for packaging into frozen fish products). Most of these are crumbed in soy flour and pre-fried in seed oils. Most of the polyunsaturated fat in those products is omega-6 from the oils and coatings. Products that claim to be 100 per cent fish (such as the Birds Eye Natural Salmon Fillet) are the obvious exception.

Clearly, crumbing and frying the fish yourself is the best way to minimise your exposure to omega-6 fats (as long as you choose the correct fish – see the table above). But some of the frozen-food options can be handy time-savers. Anything in the list above with less than 2.5 grams of polyunsaturated fat per 100 grams should do the trick, but it's best not to make this an everyday treat. A typical serving of fish is about 200 grams, which means you'll consume most of your daily allowance of polyunsaturated fats in one serving (especially if you have chips too).

We used to have fish and chips from the local shop every Friday night. I shudder to think how much seed oil we were wolfing down in that one weekly sitting. Obviously we now make our own, but that requires quite a bit of effort. I know I say most things about assembling food are easier than you think, but crumbing fish fillets and then deep-frying them (there's a recipe for this in *Toxic Oil*) isn't one of them. This means we now have fish and chips an awful lot less than we used to, and when we do have it, it's an extra-special treat. Oddly, that sort of feels right. It shouldn't be something you eat all the time. It *is* a treat.

Alcohol

I don't think I've ever spoken to anyone about quitting sugar and not have them ask me about alcohol. The number-one question for most people is 'Does this mean I have to give up the booze?' The answer is no, but you do need to be selective, and if weight loss is your goal then hitting the turps won't help. Alcoholic drinks are made by turning sugars into ethanol. As a result, very little of the sugar in, say, grape juice is left by the time you have wine. Even the sweetest dessert wines are only around 4 per cent sugar.

I've listed the best alcoholic drink choices in the 'Shopping list' at the end of the book, but in summary, use your tastebuds to guide your wine selection – a wine that tastes sweet contains sugar and should be avoided. Don't mix hard liquor with sugar (à la whiskey and coke), ciders should be avoided and beer is generally okay.

It is, however, worth noting that while alcohol isn't part of a sugar addiction, it is, of course, addictive in its own right. The other important thing to note about alcohol is that it, too, causes a significant increase in fat production and storage. Indeed, sugar is almost as efficient at creating circulating fat after it's fermented to ethanol as it is before. Drinking alcohol and eating sugar will result in some of the diseases caused by sugar (such as gout, kidney disease and liver disease) appearing more quickly than if you were just an alcoholic or sugarholic. This is because you're layering occasional (fat-creating) alcohol consumption on top of minute-by-minute (fat-creating) fructose consumption. And even if you're sugar-free, some worrying new research suggests that the presence of omega-6 polyunsaturated fats in cell membranes accelerates the neuronal death (brain damage) caused by binge drinking (at least in rats).

While some of the disease outcomes are similar, the science suggests it would be a mistake to assume that alcohol and sugar have the same effects. The body treats ethanol like any other food rather than in the special way it treats fructose. Your body will count any alcohol you drink as food, so in that sense it's not like fructose at all. Alcohol calories count, and, as long as you haven't broken your appetite-control system with fructose, it will be difficult to eat much else if booze is a big part of your diet. That's not to say you should go on an all-alcohol diet. It's addictive, and its addictive nature can cause you to overconsume it. If you drink it in serious quantities on a frequent basis, there's no doubt that you'll suffer much of the damage you'd otherwise do with fructose.

But the occasional alcoholic drink won't do any significant damage once you've eliminated the added fructose from your diet. Some research even suggests that small amounts will actually assist with arterial health. If, however, you consume grog at the rate the average person consumes fructose (up to 100 grams per day – approximately twenty standard drinks per day), then you'll merely have swapped one deadly addiction for another.

If you restrict yourself to one standard drink
(5 grams of ethanol) per day you should
be fine once you're fructose-free.

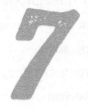

EATING OUT

Most of us need to rely on others to cook for us quite a bit of the time. We may not be hanging out at the local five–Michelin Star French restaurant on a nightly basis, but we do often need to buy lunch on the run. Some of us even occasionally get invited

---

THE EATING-OUT RULES OF THUMB

1. **If it's sweet, don't eat:** The best thing about fructose is that you can taste it. If a food or drink tastes sweet, someone has been adding sugar – avoid it.
2. **If it's fried, don't touch it:** Fried food in Australia has probably been fried in seed oil.
3. **Avoid condiments:** The sauces are full of sugar and the dressings are full of seed oil. Order your bacon and egg sarny without the barbecue sauce, your salad without the balsamic vinegar and your chicken sandwich without the mayo.

out to restaurants (that don't feature a red-headed clown). It's almost impossible to go through every option you might have available and provide guidance on what to choose, but I can give some guidelines and some advice for some of the more common options. First off, here are three handy rules of thumb.

Follow those rules and you can't go wrong, but if you want a little more detail, keep reading.

Fried food

Unless you're very, very lucky, you won't be able to purchase food fried in anything but seed oils in Australia. The 'healthy fats' message propagated by the Australian Heart Foundation has infiltrated all the major fast-food chains and every corner store. You can assume therefore, unless you know otherwise, that any frying has occurred in seed oil. Some businesses cater to the growing demand for lard in the deep-fryer (for example, 98 Fish on Queensland's Sunshine Coast), and I do my best to keep an up-to-date map of them all in my free online database (davidgillespie.org/business_map – or just go to davidgillespie.org and choose 'Business reviews' from the 'Free tools' menu). See more about this database below.

McDonald's is one of the few fast-food joints that publish comprehensive listings of their ingredients and nutrition information, so it's a handy guide to what you're likely to find in the carton at most other places. Even better, there's some handy historical data on fat breakdowns. I've shown an interesting before and after breakdown in the chart below. In 2004, McDonald's changed from frying in tallow (beef fat) to using a seed oil. The chart illustrates the dramatic effect that had on the polyunsaturated-fat content of their fries. A large fries has gone from something you could eat and easily keep within your omega-6 budget (because it contained just 1 gram of the dangerous fat) to something that knocks off your whole budget in one go and gives you even more (7 grams).

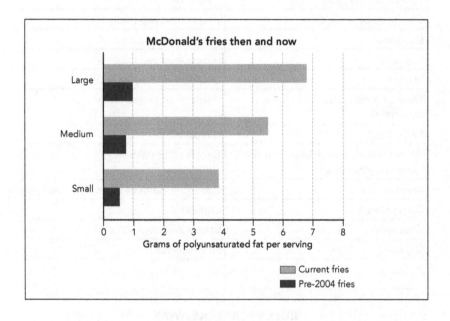

Even if you completely avoid the fried food at Macca's, you still won't be avoiding omega-6 fats. Here's a few of their non-fried foods containing seed oils.

Menu item	Oil used
Buns (including sourdough rolls and muffins but not breakfast bagels)	Canola oil
Big Mac sauce	Soybean oil (primary ingredient)
Mayonnaise	Soybean oil (primary ingredient)
Seared breast fillet	Sunflower oil (last ingredient)
Barbecue sauce	Soybean oil

Menu item	Oil used
Hollandaise-style sauce	Unspecified vegetable oil (primary ingredient)
Chocolate birthday cake	Soybean oil and palm-kernel oil
Hotcakes	Canola oil
Sausage patty (in breakfast muffins)	Canola oil
Soft-serve cone (just the cone)	Canola oil
Chocolate brownie slice	Unspecified vegetable fat
Doughnut	Palm oil and soybean oil
Cupcake	Unspecified vegetable oil
Scones	Unspecified vegetable oil
Choc caramel croissant (in the chocolate)	Unspecified vegetable oil
Raisin toast	Canola oil
White and wholemeal breads (used in toasted sandwiches)	Canola oil or palm oil
Muffins	Canola oil, palm oil and cottonseed oil
Carrot cake	Canola oil
Cheesecake	Unspecified vegetable oil
Soy milk	Sunflower oil

RULES FOR TAKEAWAY

- The only suitable drinks are unflavoured coffee, tea, water and milk. Diet drinks are okay if you really must, but probably not a good thing to get in the habit of buying (see my detailed analysis of why in *The Sweet Poison Quit Plan*).
- Stay away from the fried food unless you know what kind of oil is used.
- Obviously, any kind of dessert, muffin or cake is out.
- Ask for your meal to be made without added sauce, dressing or mayo unless you know the ingredients.

There won't be much seed oil in most of the things on this list. The point of presenting it is to give you a feel for how pervasive seed oils have become. Barely anything sold in a fast-food restaurant will be completely free of seed oils. It's best to know this going in, and do your utmost to avoid as much of it as you can – perhaps just have a nice cheap flat white (without flavouring) and eat a sandwich when you get home.

Pizza

In the average pizza shop, the danger doesn't lurk in the fryer (mainly because there isn't one), but pizzas aren't a polyunsaturated-fat-free zone. All major chains now use seed oils in their bases and in some of their toppings. Here's a representative sample provided to me by Pizza Hut:

- Soybean oil is used in the Deep Pan, Perfecto, Mia, Thin 'n Crispy and Stuffed Crust pizza bases.
- The ingredients list for the gluten-free base simply states 'vegetable oil' and doesn't specify the source.
- The pans on which the pizzas are baked are oiled with soybean oil.
- The beef topping contains canola oil.
- The chicken topping contains cottonseed oil.
- The olives are drained from a mix of olive, soybean and sunflower seed oils.
- The beef meatballs contain canola oil.
- The garlic breads contain canola oil.

All of that adds up (using the 'Fats and oils cheat sheet' in Chapter 6) to about 2 grams of polyunsaturated fat per pizza for a thin base, 4 grams for a medium base and 6 grams for a deep (pan) base. Eat a whole pizza and you've blown your polyunsaturated fat budget for the day, but you can certainly get away with a few slices every now and then.

On top of that, you'll also be getting some sugar from the sauce and the toppings, around half a teaspoon's worth per slice (and up to a whole teaspoon for the average Hawaiian). Half a pizza (1–3 grams of polyunsaturated fat and 2–4 teaspoons of sugar) won't kill you, but it's not something you want to be eating every day, either. Garlic bread is the pizza joint's equivalent of 'Do you want fries with that?' Like most commercial breads, they are made with canola oil and will add about 1 gram of polyunsaturated fat per 100 grams to your meal.

Frozen pizzas seem to be made with similar amounts of oil. But sugar is a different matter. For some reason they are loaded with the stuff.

Avoid frozen pizzas – they have up to five times the sugar content of takeaways.

A good option for pizza is to make it yourself. I've provided Lizzie's foolproof pizza dough recipe in Chapter 10 and a sauce recipe to go with it. All you need is a taste for pizza, whatever real-food ingredients you want to chuck on top and 10 minutes in a very hot oven.

If you want an even easier path, you can use frozen pizza bases. McCain's are a little high in sugar (3.6 grams per base) but have very little polyunsaturated fat. If you're after gluten-free, then either use corn or rice flour in the recipe or buy the excellent frozen bases (which seem to have no added oil or sugar at all) from Naturally Glutenfree.

Asian foods

Most of us encounter Asian foods at our local corner restaurant. The food is usually cooked according to the whim of the owner, and the nutrition content is neither measured nor published. This makes it almost impossible to provide guidance on what to eat in the same way I have elsewhere, but I'll give it a go.

Some chain restaurants specialise in Asian cuisines, and some of those do publish their nutrition content. Noodle Box is one

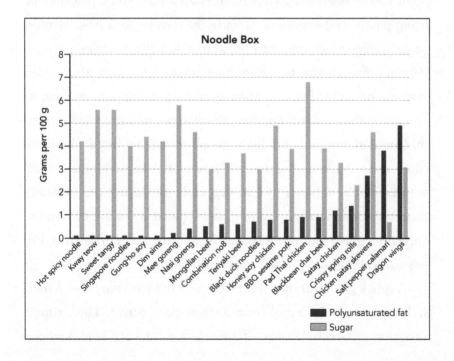

such outfit. It has some great choices that are extremely low in polyunsaturated fat. Unfortunately, they all contain more than a teaspoon of sugar in every 100 grams (which is four teaspoons even in a small box).

The best choices are those with very little polyunsaturated fat and a lower sugar content. At Noodle Box, these are the Pad Thai Chicken, the Kway Teow and the Nasi Goreng. Since a small serving of any of these foods is around 400 grams and a large is around 700 grams, most of them contain huge doses of sugar. A small Pad Thai Chicken, for example, has almost 28 grams (seven teaspoons) of sugar, and a large contains almost 49 grams (twelve teaspoons). The prawn crackers and spring rolls are deep-fried in seed oil, and must be avoided completely because of their very high polyunsaturated-fat content.

If you're assembling your own Asian foods, you'll probably be using pastes and sauces to provide the flavour to a base of meat or fish, vegetables and carbohydrates (usually noodles or rice). Rice is a fine choice as a meal base because it has neither added seed oil nor added sugar. Most noodles are fine too, as long as you avoid the 'instant' noodles, which are often pre-fried in seed oil (check the ingredients list – no oil should be listed). If you're using a kit (such as Marion's Kitchen or Asia at Home), you'll see that you're advised to add vegetable oil during the assembly process. Simply change that to olive oil (or, if you want to be more authentic, ghee) and you'll be fine from a seed-oil perspective, but pay careful attention to the sugar content.

A quick glance at the table below will tell you that some Asian-style sauces can be lethal from a sugar perspective. There's huge variation between brands of like-named sauces. For example,

Chang's hoisin (7.1 per cent) has about a fifth the sugar of Ayam's hoisin (35.3 per cent). But Kikkoman's teriyaki (12.6 per cent) has about a third the sugar of the Masterfoods version (36.3 per cent). There are many more brands than the sample below, so it's definitely worth looking for a different brand if one of your favourites scores badly on this list. Most Asian recipes don't call for huge amounts of these sauces, so you can probably safely use most of the ones above the Kikkoman teriyaki in this table.

Brand	Sauce	% sugar
Yeo's	Sesame Oil	—
Pandaroo	Sesame Oil	—
Ayam	Fish	0.50
Kikkoman	Soy	1.30
Squid Brand	Fish	1.30
Empower Foods	LC Satay (contains sucralose)	1.50
Kikkoman	Gluten Free Soy	1.90
Kikkoman	Organic Soy	2.30
Chang's	Dark Soy	3.30
Empower Foods	LC Sweet & Sour (contains sucralose)	3.70
Kikkoman	Tamari Soy	3.90
Kikkoman	Less Salt Soy	5.10
Masterfoods	Homestyle Thai	4.20
Masterfoods	Soy	4.30
Maggi	Fish	6.00
Chang's	Light Soy	6.20
Hakubaku	Chilli Soy Noodle	6.40
Chang's	Fish	6.70
Chang's	Hoisin	7.10
Chang's	Ponzu	8.80
Kikkoman	Sushi & Sashimi Soy	9.60
Pandaroo	Sushi Soy	9.60
Pandaroo	Sushi Vinegar	9.60

Brand	Sauce	% sugar
Chang's	Oyster	9.70
Chang's	Pure Sesame Oil	9.70
Chang's	Tasty Sichuan Stir Fry	10.20
Chang's	Black bean	11.00
Ayam	Soya	11.20
Chang's	Spicy Sichuan Stir Fry	12.00
Kikkoman	Teriyaki	12.60
Kikkoman	Teriyaki Hot 'n' Spicy	13.70
Ayam	Black bean	17.30
Woolworths	Select Oriental Soy Garlic & Honey	20.20
Kikkoman	Roasted Garlic & Soy	20.90
Ayam	Vegetarian Stir-Fry	21.10
Makubaku	Wasabi Noodle	21.30
Fountain	Satay	22.30
Masterfoods	Satay	23.10
Ayam	Japanese Black Sesame Dressing	23.50
Beerenberg	Huey's Teriyaki Grill	24.00
Woolworths	Select Singapore Satay	24.20
Ayam	Vietnamese Tangy Dressing	24.30
Ayam	Thai Ginger Sesame Dressing	24.30
Ayam	Oyster	26.50
Masterfoods	Soy, Sesame & Ginger	26.70
Kikkoman	Japanese BBQ	27.10
Kikkoman	Sesame Ginger & Soy	28.80
Ayam	Mongolian Lamb	30.20
Ayam	Plum	30.40
Masterfoods	Sweet & Sour	32.30
Ayam	Honey & Soy	32.30
Pandaroo	Sushi Seasoning	32.90
Kikkoman	Sweet Chilli, Ginger and Soy	34.00
Kikkoman	Sweet Soy	35.30
Ayam	Hoi Sin	35.30
Poonsin	Vietnamese Dipping	35.60
Masterfoods	Soy, Honey & Garlic	35.80

Brand	Sauce	% sugar
McDonalds	Sweet & Sour	35.80
Masterfoods	Teriyaki	36.30
Beerenberg	Taka Tala	40.00
Ayam	Teriyaki	42.90
Ayam	Vietnamese Dipping Sauce	43.90
Ayam	Sweet & Sour	46.20
Ayam	Lemon Chicken	47.60
Kikkoman	Honey & Soy	53.20
Ayam	San Choy Bao	54.70
Ayam	Thick Soya	63.90

The good news is that none of these sauces, with the exception of the sesame seed oil, contains any appreciable amount of polyunsaturated fat. Unfortunately, sesame seed oil is 44 per cent polyunsaturated fat and should be avoided for anything other than flavouring with very small quantities. In place of sesame oil, you can use any of the 'safe' fats and oils I set out in the table on page 118, but you'll miss out on that sesame seed taste. The best way to simulate it is to use a cooking oil that doesn't have much flavour (such as refined olive oil) and throw in some whole sesame seeds for flavour.

This doesn't mean you have to avoid Asian food. You just need to be careful. In Australia, the vast majority of it is cooked in seed oils and many of the sauces contain significant amounts of sugar. The following rules of thumb might help. But as always, remember: if you know how the food is being cooked, then you'll always be well ahead of the game.

It is, of course, possible (and easy) to make most Asian dishes from scratch using ingredients that contain no (or minimal) sugar or seed oil. Give it a go – it's fun (and, with the money you save, you could take yourself on an Asian holiday instead).

In cooking your own, be careful of shortcuts. Curry pastes are usually made with seed oils. Use curry powder instead, or go the whole hog and do the flavours from scratch. In about a second and a half of internet searching you should be able to discover thousands of recipes for homemade curry. If any call for seed oils (rice bran seems to be a favourite in many), just use olive oil instead.

Mexican food

Mexican food rarely contains added seed oil, but it's often seasoned with sauces that are loaded with sugar. In the chart below, I've lined up, in order of ascending sugar content, most of the major brands selling products you'd use in assembling a Mexican dish at home.

The best soft wraps are Old El Paso Wholegrain Tortillas or the Mission White Corn Tortillas. Old El Paso looks to be the best choice for hard taco shells. They're made using the modified high-oleic sunflower oil (see page 164) rather than standard sunflower or canola oil. And while they still have a relatively high oil content, bear in mind that 100 grams of taco shells is nine standard tacos. So unless you really pig out, you won't be doing a whole lot of damage to your daily allowance of omega-6 fats. Under no circumstances go anywhere near the reduced-salt taco shell – it's practically confectionery.

The seasonings are where these manufacturers really load up on the sugar. It's beyond me why a fajita seasoning needs to be almost half sugar. The best choice (of a bad lot) is the Old El Paso Burrito seasoning.

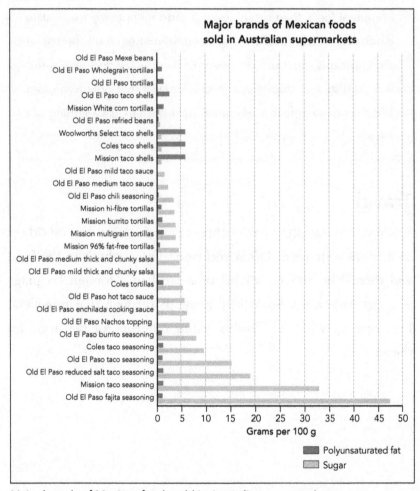

Major brands of Mexican foods sold in Australian supermarkets

Travel

When you're travelling you're almost entirely dependent on others to prepare your food. Often you won't know what's in the food and there'll be either no label or a label in a foreign language (such as American). So to help guide us through that minefield, I've come up with the 'Twelve commandments for real food on the go'.

THE TWELVE COMMANDMENTS FOR REAL FOOD ON THE GO

1. Assume everything an airline or restaurant attempts to serve you is fake food – eat it, but be careful and apply commandments 2–7.
2. Avoid all condiments and sauces.
3. Avoid all packaged breakfast cereals.
4. Drink only water, milk, tea, coffee and alcohol (if you wish).
5. Avoid anything else that tastes sweet.
6. Avoid anything that's fried (unless you know what it's fried in).
7. Ask for butter instead of margarine.
8. Buy your daily bread from a baker, not a shopkeeper.
9. Don't stress about whether the meat is grass-fed (but choose it if you can).
10. Purchase fresh rather than packaged food.
11. Make your own sandwiches.
12. If possible, book accommodation that's self-cook (apartments) rather than a hotel room.

WHAT TO EXPECT WHEN QUITTING SUGAR

Unfortunately, shopping and cooking are the easy bits of deciding to eat real food. When you first start out you'll also be dealing with a nasty little catch to the whole thing. You'll need to break your sugar addiction. I know you don't think you have one – neither did I. But after just a few days of eating real food you'll feel like you've been dragged backwards through a garbage dump. You'll have headaches, mood swings and irresistible cravings for your old favourites (such as chocolate). At that point you may well say to yourself, 'This real-food caper leaves a lot to be desired.' But that's not the real food doing the damage, it's you going through withdrawal from sugar. This section is designed to prepare you for that and provide some tips for getting through it. I can't pretend it will be easy, because for most people it isn't. But it's well and truly worth it. When you emerge from the other side, you'll be free from your food addiction and free to enjoy the real taste of real food and the real health that flows from eating it. The following pointers are a summary of a much more detailed description laid out in *The Sweet Poison Quit Plan*. If you still have questions about how to rid yourself of sugar after reading this, then I recommend you take a look at the more detailed version.

Addiction

We don't have the word 'chocoholic' in the language because cocoa is addictive. Raw cocoa is slightly less tasty than dirt. But when we add sugar, suddenly magic happens. You know as well as I do sugar is addictive. To prove it, I could point you to a pile of studies you couldn't jump over but there's an easier (and more convincing) way to do it. Stop. That's right, just totally eliminate sugar from your life for seven days and see how you feel. Spoiler alert: You'll feel like crap. Indeed many ex-smokers tell me they felt exactly the same giving up sugar as when they quit the fags, only with sugar it was worse. This is no ordinary food. Ordinary food doesn't make you feel terrible when you stop eating it. If I asked you to stop eating broccoli for seven days, you'd barely notice it (believe me, I can do so with ease). Even if broccoli was your favourite food in the whole world, you might feel a bit sad, but you wouldn't feel like you were going through withdrawal from nicotine.

You can know everything there is to know about the nasty things sugar will do to you, but until you understand that you're an addict, you won't change your behaviour. Worse than that, your addictive substance of choice has been added to almost every food on the supermarket shelf. You're gonna need some help.

Make no mistake: the task you're about to undertake won't be easy, but it's not an exercise in willpower. Just like willpower-based methods of quitting smoking, diets don't work. You can't overcome a chemical addiction with willpower (see page 94 for the detail on why).

You're not a glutton. You're not weak-willed. You're chemically addicted to a substance in the food supply called fructose. And until you treat that addiction as the powerful biochemical force it is, you'll never loosen its grip.

Losing your sugar addiction

There are five steps to beating your addiction.

Step 1: Have the right attitude

When you have a cigarette or strong coffee or suck on a sweet, your reward system lights up. You feel good, even if only momentarily. You feel more alive, sharper, more capable. This is the serotonin–dopamine cycle (see Chapter Two) at work and it's what drives addiction. The good feelings don't last forever. Soon enough you'll be feeling less capable, less smart and less able to cope. It's not your imagination, that's the dip that pays for the dopamine spike. But not to worry, you can fix it with another hit. Sadly, the research on addiction tells us that that next hit will require just a little bit more of the addictive substance to deliver the same value as the first. We become inured and need more and more just to feel good again. An addict swings from feeling good to feeling bad like a pendulum. The trouble is that even when they feel good they don't feel as good as the non-addict feels all the time.

It's an extreme example but picture a heroin addict alternating between mindless euphoria and the desperate search for the next hit. Do you really want to be that poor wretch (with a more socially acceptable drug)? Once you understand that you're breaking a cycle of addiction rather than going on a diet, it becomes much easier to stay on track. You won't wish you were eating the chocolate cake being passed around at morning tea because you'll no longer wish to be an addict. You'll be no more envious of the addicts eating the cake than you would be of the heroin addict. You'll understand that if you did have a piece you'd momentarily feel good but then the cycle of addiction would start all over again and feeling bad would be just around the corner. Stay the path and you'll feel good all the time. You're not dieting, you're quitting. It's an important mindset to lock in right from the start. And every day you manage it is a day closer to not wanting the sugar at all.

Step 2: Identify your sugar-eating habits

Habits reinforce addictive behaviour. Before I quit sugar I'd relax in the evening in front of the telly (six kids can be exhausting). Part of that ritual was to have a sweet treat of some sort, maybe a bit of chocolate or a Mint Slice biscuit (or three) or even some ice-cream. The relaxing part was sitting in front of the telly getting to do (and think) nothing. But sugar got the credit. It had become a part of that relaxation, such that it would feel strange to do it without the sugar. Sugar infiltrates our pleasurable habits in that way and makes it seem like an inextricable component. As you're about to discover, that simply isn't true. Once you break your sugar addiction, you can still pursue your pleasurable habits and, believe it or not, they'll be just as much fun without the sugar. But in the meantime, having sugar bound up with pleasure in that way is going to make it difficult to get sugar out of your life. To do it, you need to know what your sugar-pleasure habits are and change them until you successfully delete sugar. The best thing to do is make a list. Be thorough. Leave no stone unturned. This is a critical part of breaking your addiction.

Here's my list from my pre-sugar-free life.

MY LIST OF HABITS BEFORE I BROKE MY SUGAR ADDICTION

1. Every time I have a cup of tea (which could be five or six times a day), I accompany it with a biscuit (or three).
2. I always have a juice with breakfast.
3. I always look forward to a dessert after dinner.
4. I always eat a few pieces of chocolate in front of the TV at night. On weekends, this might extend to a chocolate-coated ice-cream.
5. If I'm buying a coffee, I get myself a blueberry muffin to go with it.
6. When out shopping, I can't walk past a vending machine without acquiring a soft drink.
7. When I'm at McDonald's, I always order the 'meal deal' with a soft drink because it's easier (and probably cheaper). And I finish off the meal by visiting the counter again for a soft-serve cone.

Put the book down right now and make your list. Go on, do it. Be brutally honest. You don't need to show it to anyone (unless you plan to write a book, I guess), but make sure it's complete. In your mind, walk through a typical day and think about how and when you're exposed to sugar and what triggers that exposure.

Step 3: Eliminate those habits

Now that you know when you're likely to be confronted by the desire to chow down on sugar, you can come up with a plan for dealing with it or avoiding the situation altogether. My list of avoidance strategies looked like this:

MY LIST OF AVOIDANCE STRATEGIES

1. Keep a jar of nuts by the kettle and remove the bickies. That way I can still have a snack when I have a cuppa, but sugar won't be an option.
2. Substitute milk or water for fruit juice with breakfast.
3. Remove all sugar-containing dessert ingredients from the house. Enjoy a non-sugar treat (perhaps some potato crisps) after dinner.

4. Substitute nuts for chocolate for my TV-watching snack.

5. When I buy a coffee, choose a non-sugar accompaniment (like buttered thick toast). If the establishment doesn't offer a non-sugar option, choose a different coffee purveyor.

6. When I spot a vending machine while out shopping, choose a bottled water or a diet drink instead of a full-strength soft drink.

7. At McDonald's, substitute diet soft drink in the 'meal deal' and ditch the after-meal treat.

8. If I exercise, give myself a non-food-based reward: shout myself to the movies or drop by the video library on the way home (but see also points 4 and 9).

9. Switch to diet soft drinks at the movies.

10. Switch to diet drinks when out or just drink (unflavoured) mineral water.

11. Switch to a diet tonic water in my G and T.

It might seem silly that I'm making you write these things out, but it's worth the bother. In making the list you're forced to think carefully about exactly what you'll do. When you're confronted with a sudden desire for a muffin at the coffee counter, what's your plan? Writing down 'I'll order hot buttered toast' forces you to concoct a plan and makes sure you remember your plan when the situation actually arises. Sometimes the only viable plan is to avoid the situation altogether. If you can't face going to the movies without Maltesers then just skip the movies until you're through withdrawal. It won't be long before you can go again and (as I do now) look in wonder at the room full of people who can't get through 90 minutes without eating their weight in sweets – oh, and watching a movie.

This may not be a complete list. Things change and you might also have missed something. If you encounter a new sugar-filled situation, don't hesitate to add it to the list and work out an appropriate avoidance strategy. And even though this might all seem a bit heavy-handed just to avoid sugar, believe me, it helps. Having a plan means you won't be easily lured into thoughtless sugar consumption. Soon enough you'll be through withdrawal and you won't even give sugar a second thought, but in the meantime, make the lists.

Methadone for sugar addicts

I'm often asked about artificial sweeteners. My answer is to treat them like methadone for sugar addicts. Use them to get off the gear but don't use them in the long term. I don't know whether they'll be safe in 50 years time, and neither does anyone else. There are too many deep pockets funding both sides of the science on sweeteners (the sugar industry on one side and the sweetener makers on the other) to be confident in science that says there's nothing to worry about. The good news is that you probably won't want to keep consuming them after withdrawal anyway. As you go through withdrawal, your palate adjusts quite considerably. Sweeteners that taste a lot like sugar at the beginning will taste like chemical cocktails by the end. Most people don't find them too hard to give up.

> **Only sugar addicts think sugar substitutes taste like sugar.**

If you want to read more detail on what we know about each of the sugar substitutes, how our body handles them and how dangerous they might or might not be, I recommend you take a look at the relevant section in *The Sweet Poison Quit Plan.*

Step 4: Get your house in order

You'd never quit smoking if you had a house full of cigarettes, and you'll never quit sugar if you have a house full of food containing it. So this is the bit where you rummage through your cupboards and fridge, replacing all your sugar- and seed-oil-filled fake food with real food. Use the guides in Chapter 6 and it should be easy-peasy. Once you're done, come back to the book for Step 5.

Step 5: Withdrawal

I'm not going to sugar-coat it for you. Withdrawal from sugar addiction isn't fun. But it's not terrible either, and the rewards are well and truly worth it. The key is to make a conscious start. Set a time and a date when it's going to happen and determinedly start. From 9 am Monday morning (for example) you won't knowingly consume sugar ever again. There's no point going down the eating-in-moderation route (what does that even mean anyway?). You can't stop smoking by only having ten ciggies a day and you can't quit sugar by cutting your cupcake allowance in half. You're either eating sugar or you're not. So make sure that from that time onwards, you're not.

What will withdrawal be like?

Everybody notices feeling different and most people say it's like coming down with a bad flu. You feel headachy, hungry or thirsty most of the time and generally under the weather. It doesn't hurt (much) but it's no barrel of laughs, either.

At the start you'll probably feel like eating all the time. Even if you're not hungry you'll still feel like a snack. This is how sugar cravings feel. Your body knows, through many years of hard training, that the best way to get some sugar is to make you feel hungry (or thirsty). I suggest just going with it – eat. Have loads of sugar-free snacks on hand (I bought a case of Pepsi Max and loaded it into the fridge). Make them things you like – expensive salted nuts or creamy soft cheese or whatever it is that floats your boat (without sugar). If they're high-fat snacks then so much the better, you'll fill up quickly. Often people who think quitting sugar is a diet fret about all the fat they'll be consuming in this phase and worry they'll be piling on the pounds. Sometimes they do, but this is no time for trying to abstain. You're breaking a strong addiction and now isn't the time to beat yourself up. This phase will be over soon enough.

Around three days in, the headaches will stop and so too will the hunger. Your addicted brain is starting to come to the realisation that you won't be caving in. Most people report that at this stage they felt no desire for food at all. They could have gone all day and not even noticed that they hadn't eaten. But just because you're not hungry doesn't mean you can't be tempted. Keep your avoidance strategies handy; you'll need them.

Over the next few weeks your appetite should slowly start to return to normal, but it won't be like it was before. You'll start to notice that you suddenly feel full (to the point of nausea) before you get to the end of a meal you would have polished off easily before. You'll also notice that when you're hungry you're really hungry ('Feed me now or I'll eat this desk' hungry). It will feel different from the pseudo-hunger you felt at the start of withdrawal. That wasn't real hunger that was your addicted brain trying to simulate hunger. Now you'll know what hunger is really like. The other thing you'll notice is that, having eaten, you'll stay satisfied for much longer than you did before. When I was a sugar addict I would chow down on my bowl of Heart Foundation–approved Just Right for breakfast and by mid-morning I'd be starving – which was always a good excuse for elevenses. Now, I'll eat a sausage and egg (one of each) and not feel hungry again until lunchtime or even dinnertime. Suddenly you'll find yourself no longer needing snacks. You'll be fine with three square meals a day (or even less).

This phase is the least predictable. Some people don't look back after a week off the gear, others find themselves dreaming about chocolate sundaes up to a year later. It's different for everyone (and anecdotally harder and longer for women), but one thing you should know for certain is that every day you'll be less drawn to sugar than you were the day before. And then suddenly, one day someone offers you a free chocolate and you just say no without a moment's thought. Magic! Welcome to the rest of your life.

The good news: seed oils aren't addictive

Seed oils are just fat in another form. They're designed to be identical in mouthfeel and use to the fats we cooked with for generations. Getting them out of your diet will be done on autopilot if you follow the guides set out in Chapter Six. Once you're eating real food, you're automatically no longer eating seed oils. Even better than that, there's no addiction element to deal with. So switching to real fat is as easy as knowing what you're eating. Real food made with real fat and without sugar tastes better than any fake food you've ever eaten. You'll never look back.

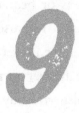

THE PRACTICAL BIT

How to shop for and store food

This may seem like a section designed to state the bleedin' obvious, but since the 1980s, home economics has been progressively eliminated from the school curriculum. There are now several generations of us who don't have the first clue what to buy or how to store real food. If you do, then feel free to skip to the next bit. If not, keep reading – your secret disability is safe with me.

Fruit and vegetables

One of the biggest problems with fruit and veg is it tends to go off if you don't eat it, so many of us spend a fair chunk of money feeding the bin. The solution is to get very precise about what you actually use, or discover the wonders of the freezer section of the supermarket. Frozen vegetables are every bit as good for you as the fresh kind. And there's absolutely nothing wrong (and quite a lot right, when it comes to price) with buying your broccoli, carrots, peas or beans snap-frozen. It also cuts down enormously on waste. You use what you need and put the rest back in the freezer for next time. Sure, it's good to eat fresh, but if you have the freezer to rely on you can get meal-specific about anything else you buy. For example, we always have a proper family roast (beef, usually) once a week. For that, we always buy fresh. But we know exactly what we'll need for that meal and shop for exactly that, no more, no less. Since I'm the shopper (well, on the weekends anyway) I can reveal our secret ingredients: eight whole potatoes (for baking), 1 kilogram of carrots, two broccoli heads (a quarter head per person), one sweet potato and four corn cobs (half per person). Not one thing will be wasted from that lot because that's exactly what will end up on the plate.

When it comes to fruit, frozen is really only an option for berries. It's a very good option, mind you. They're usually significantly cheaper and, when thawed, significantly nicer than the ones you can get fresh, plus, once again, there's no waste. But if a banana is what you desire, then a frozen blueberry won't cut the mustard. Whole fresh fruit should be counted precisely and purchased accurately. At our place we know that four of our kids are going to want an apple one day, a banana the next and a kiwifruit the day after. So we buy four of each once a week. With about two minutes planning you can probably come up with an accurate estimate of your weekly fruit needs too.

If you're buying whole fresh fruit and vegetables, here are ten things everyone should know about fresh fruit and veg:

1. Store potatoes and onions in a cool, dry, dark place – a kitchen cabinet or the pantry are good spots.

2. Buy brown onions rather than white or red – they're much cheaper and look the same once cooked. Only get red onions if you're trying to add colour to a salad.

3. Wash all fruit when you get it home. Store fruit (including tomatoes) out of the fridge until ripe and then put it in the fridge to stop the ripening. A banana's skin will go brown in the fridge, but that doesn't mean it's gone off. Just peel it and you're good to go (although you'll never convince a child of that, so peel it before you give it to them).

4. Stone fruit goes off much more quickly than apples and pears – keep an eye on it.

5. Store watermelon in the fridge unless you plan to eat it immediately – it's sold ripe.

6. Whole pineapple is fine out of the fridge until you cut into it, then it should be refrigerated.

7. Store avocados in a paper bag to ripen them (they're slightly soft to the touch when ripe, but rock-hard before that) and then put them in the fridge.

8. All fresh vegetables (except potatoes) last longest in the fresh-food drawer (crisper) in the fridge.

9. Wash lettuce as soon as you buy it and store it in the fridge (preferably in one of those round plastic lettuce-storers that keep them out of the water at the bottom of the container).

10. Don't expect fruit to last longer than a week or vegetables longer than two weeks.

Meat

You should assume that all meat sold in a supermarket is lot-fed (see Chapter 6 for why this matters), although as I explained earlier, that's not necessarily a bad thing. If, however, you do decide to stick to grass-fed meat, you'll find that it's not impossible or even outrageously expensive. I maintain a free online database (see davidgillespie.org/product_list) of local farmers who supply the increasing demand for free-range meat.

A recent addition to the Australian retail scene is Aldi, and blow me down if it doesn't have a grass-fed meat section. The Aldi range, which covers everything from fillet steak to mince, only costs a little more than the lot-fed options it also sells. If you don't have an Aldi nearby, try your local butcher. Almost all their meat will be lot-fed but they can probably get you grass-fed meat if you give them some notice. Don't assume that just because meat is displayed in a window it's any different from the shrink-wrapped stuff at Woolies.

There are no special storage instructions for meat other than to keep it in the fridge until just before you cook it. If the use-by date is fast approaching and you know you won't get to it, chuck it in the freezer. That will give you more time (a few more months) to use it.

It's a good idea to thaw frozen meat (by leaving it out on the sink until defrosted or just using a microwave) before you start cooking it. Otherwise it will likely be quite tough to chew. When you cook a roast (chicken, beef, lamb or pork), choose a size bigger than you need for that meal. The leftover cooked meat makes great ready-to-go filling for sandwiches for the rest of the week. And in general, think leftovers (by cooking extra) whenever you cook. Many things are just as good the second time round, and if all it needs is a quick reheat, you've created your own version of convenience food.

Store eggs in the fridge from the moment you get them home. If you do this, the use-by date isn't critical. Believe me, it's very easy to tell when an egg is off. The smell is unbearable.

Butter

Store butter in the fridge until you plan to use it. Butter can be left out of the fridge for a week (depending on the temperature) because its fats are predominately animal fats and they don't easily oxidise (go rancid). How much and how long you leave it out depends on your usage patterns and the ambient temperature. Butter is rock-hard at 4°C (the temperature of the average fridge), almost spreadable at 15°C (Melbourne daytime winter temperature), perfect at 23°C (Brisbane daytime winter temperature) and a puddle at 33°C (Darwin daytime temperature all year round). Salted butter lasts longer than unsalted (salt is a preservative), so we tend to buy both – salted for the bread and unsalted for the cooking. You'll know if your butter has gone rancid because it will turn a darker shade of yellow and taste and smell funny. Don't worry, it won't hurt you to eat it, but I wouldn't recommend it as a gastronomic experience.

We live in Brisbane and we have six kids (two of whom have now finished high school) so we go through around 500 grams of butter every few days. Most of the time we leave a butter dish (just a Pyrex dish with a rubber lid) with about that much butter in it on the kitchen counter. Some days the temperature makes it so runny you can't even get it on your knife (try spreading water and you'll get the idea). That's when we pop it in the fridge. If someone forgets to take it out, they'd better be having toast or their sandwich is going to be kinda chunky. It sounds complex, but you really do get used to it quite quickly, and before you know it you have a sixth sense for when to get the butter out of or into the fridge. You'll quickly get to know how much is a week's worth of butter at your place and get used to rotating it appropriately. Just remember to shove it in the fridge before you go on holidays.

THE FRENCH SOLUTION

Before refrigerators, the French came up with a cunning solution to the problem of oxidation. They found that if butter was stored in water, it lasted four to five times longer than if it was left exposed to air. The French butter dish is a way of storing butter in water. It consists of a pot full of water with a lid (a smaller, upside-down pot) that contains the butter. The lid is packed with butter and placed on the pot of water, completely submerging the butter in the water. As long as the water is changed regularly, a French butter pot will allow you to leave butter out of the fridge for a month or more. This will obviously be less successful in places where the butter isn't solid enough (where the room temperature is above about 27°C) to hold together when upside down.

Cooking fats

Not all fats and oils are good for cooking all things. When fats are heated past a certain temperature, they begin to smoke. This temperature is different for each fat and is called the smoke point.

The smoke is largely made up of something called acrolein. Acrolein has an acrid, piercing smell and is highly irritating to the eyes. When it's formed, the percentage of free fatty acids in the cooking fat increases dramatically. That significantly affects an oil's taste (and not in a good way), but there are no proven effects on health from consuming oil that's been heated past its smoke point, so don't be too stressed about accidentally making an oil or fat smoke.

The more free fatty acids there are, the lower the smoke point becomes. This means that if you reuse oils, each time you heat them, the smoke point becomes progressively lower. An old oil smokes more quickly than a new oil. If the oil or fat you're using is smoking, turn down the temperature straight away and consider using a different fat for the job.

In the table below, I've set out the typical smoke points for the oils you'll be using. Remember, these are rough numbers and each brand will give a slightly different result.

SMOKE POINTS OF GOOD FATS AND OILS

Temperature (°C/°F)	Fat or oil	Oven temperature	Cooking style
270/518	Refined avocado oil	Very hot	Pan-fry, wok-fry, deep-fry, use in oven
250/482	Ghee		
240/464	Extra light olive oil		
230/446	Palm oil Refined coconut oil		
220/428	Tallow (beef fat)	Hot	
210/410	Macadamia oil		
205/401	Extra virgin olive oil		
200/193	Virgin olive oil Virgin avocado oil		
190/374	Lard (pig fat)	Moderate	Deep-fry (up to 190°C/374°F)
175/347	Extra virgin coconut oil		Pan-fry or wok-fry (up to 175°C/347°F)
150–170/302–308	Butter	Slow	

In short, you can use anything to pan-fry, anything except butter or extra virgin coconut oil to deep-fry, and anything but those and lard in a hot oven.

If you're deep-frying, you'll often be able to get many meals out of the one batch of fat. It really depends what you're frying and how dirty it makes the fat. The colour of the hot fat is a guide to whether it's reusable or not. Brand-new rendered fat will be almost completely transparent or slightly golden when heated (they all look white when cooled). You should be able to see the bottom of the pan or frying pot clearly. After you use it, pour it through a strainer into a pot and keep it in the fridge until the next time you need it. As you use it for more and more fryings, it will become progressively darker. Once it's dark brown (like maple syrup) it's time to bin it. Or, if you have a dog, chop up the old cooled, solid fat for treats (which you store in the fridge) – they love it.

If olive oil is your preferred fat, store it in a dark place in a sealed container. Like all oils it breaks down when exposed to light. We buy ours in bulk tins we keep under the sink and dispense into a small bottle for table use.

The costs

We're constantly told that eating whole foods is expensive. Dietitians and health authorities constantly suggest that the reason we're all fat is that it's cheaper to eat junk. But is it? Sure, if your menu consists of wombat milk, activated bananas and (of course) goji berries, then yes, avoiding processed food will cost you an arm and a leg. But if you're practical about eating real food, it's by far the cheaper option. Here are a couple of examples.

Real food		Processed food	
Gillespie family roast (eight people)		McCain Roast Beef frozen meal (beef, potatoes, beans, carrots)	
1 kg topside beef	$14.00	8 × 320 g packets	
1 kg carrots	$2.00		
1.6 kg potatoes	$5.00		
2 broccoli	$5.00		
1 sweet potato	$2.00		
4 corn cobs	$4.00		
Total	$32.00 ($4.00 each)	Total	$60.00 ($7.50 each)
Bowl of oats (35 g)	$0.06	Bowl of Nutri-Grain (35 g)	$0.46
Coles butter (500 g)	$3.00	Margarine (500 g)	$3.00–$7.00 (depending on brand)
Coles full-fat milk (1 litre)	$1.00	Coles low-fat milk (1 litre)	$1.25

As you can see, eating real food is considerably cheaper than buying packaged food. That shouldn't come as much of a surprise. There are a lot of profit margins between you and the food when you buy it in a packet, but when you Eat Real Food, you're really only paying the farmer and the shopkeeper. And just in case you think I've been a bit selective, I've also completely costed every recipe in Chapter 10 and compared it with its processed-food alternative.

Meal planner

This section is not so much a meal planner as a meal suggester. Diet books have meal planners. They tell you what to eat for breakfast, morning tea, lunch, afternoon tea, dinner and supper for a week or even a month at a time. This isn't a diet book. It's a book that's designed to give you the tools to eat well for the rest of your life. As they say, give a man a fish and you feed him for a day, teach him to fish and you feed him for life. Prepare to learn to fish. The following sections take a detailed look at the options you'll normally encounter for each meal and give you some guidance about the choices that are likely to ensure you minimise your exposure to seed oils and sugar.

Breakfast

A modern Australian breakfast more often than not comes out of a cardboard box. And even though that packet will undoubtedly proclaim that the extruded grains within are 'ancient' or 'whole' or 'whole ancient' a serious amount of sugar will almost certainly have been added. If they didn't do that, people would almost certainly find the box more appetising than the contents. There are, however, a few exceptions to the rule. They are plain, minimally processed wheat (usually, but not always, in the form of biscuits) or rolled oats. If you look carefully in the health-food aisle you'll even find puffed rice, wheat and corn with no added sugar or oil. If in doubt, apply my sugar rule to make sure that total sugars are less than 3 grams per 100 grams and you'll be fine. There isn't a lot of seed oil in the cereal aisle except in the toasted mueslis (see 'Muesli' below), so don't worry too much about that (although it never hurts to check).

Cereals

Rolled oats are the rolled-gold choice for a sugar-free grain-based breakfast. Heat them with milk or water and you have an instant and very filling (if not terribly tasty) start to the day. If plain oats are too boring for you (or, more likely, the kids), add some berries or even a few slices of banana. Yes, they both contain fructose, but you're eating it in its original packaging so you'll be right. If you'd normally add honey to porridge, then give rice malt syrup a go. It looks like honey, tastes like honey (to people who've gone through withdrawal from sugar) but contains no fructose. Indeed, this is a good one to keep up your sleeve if you were partial to honey when you ate sugar. On any occasion you'd have added honey, try rice malt syrup instead.

If porridge is a bit boring, but you still want cereal, try wheat biscuits or oat biscuits. Most of the expensive and generic brands are at or below 3 grams of sugar per 100 grams (our lot like the Woolworths Home Brand Wheat Biscuits and then mix it up with Vita Brits every now and then). Add milk and (if you like) a sprinkle of dextrose or a drizzle of rice malt syrup or even some cut-up fruit and you have a lovely bowl of quick and easy kid fuel.

If muesli is more your speed, then Flip Shelton's Natural Muesli and The Muesli are both completely free of added fructose and seed oils. Most other mueslis add (at least) dried fruit, which significantly increases the fructose content and rules them out of contention.

WHAT'S WRONG WITH DRIED FRUIT?

When we dry fruit, we significantly concentrate the sugar. The fibre is still there but all of the bulk (largely water) associated with fruit is removed – a small box of sultanas (school lunch-box size) contains 100 sultanas (65 per cent sugar), which is the equivalent of half a kilo of Thompson seedless grapes. A child will quickly scoff down that little box and still want some morning tea, but half a kilo of grapes would slow them down significantly.

Seed oil is used to toast all commercial mueslis, so if you like the toasted variety (even if you could find one without dried fruit), your only real choice is to do it yourself. There's a very scrumptious recipe for toasted granola in *The Sweet Poison Quit Plan Cookbook*.

Toast

Check out Chapter 6 for tips on choosing the right bread. Do that right and learn to operate a toaster, and you will have an instant base for a low-seed-oil and low-sugar breakfast. If you have the time and the inclination, making your own bread guarantees it will be completely free of both (see Chapter 10 for a recipe). If you're looking for gluten-free 'toast', rice cakes are the go, but be careful – some brands use added seed oils, so check the ingredients list before purchasing.

Then, of course, you need to put something worthwhile (and non-lethal – I'm looking at you, Nutella) on the toast. My first choice would be butter. Then I would go with a poached egg. But if cooking isn't your thing, you could always smear on some Vegemite (but not Marmite – too high in sugar) or one of the safer nut butter options (see Chapter 6). Cream cheese (or any other kind of cheese, actually) is always a good option. And if you're feeling especially tropical, mash up some avocado and add in a little salt, pepper and lemon juice.

If you're really feeling fancy, toast up some homemade bruschetta, add some diced fresh tomato, capers, onion and a drizzle of olive oil, and invite me over to breakfast.

Continental breakfasts

The 'continental' breakfast usually consists of bread, butter, cheese and various cuts of meat. Well, it does in Europe. In the United States and Australia it means Danish pastries, chocolate croissants, sweetened yoghurt and (maybe) fruit salad. The European variety is a perfectly acceptable breakfast as long as you know the provenance of the bread. If it has truly been made according to traditional European bread recipes (rye, sourdough and crusty white) then it will have no added seed oil or sugar. Obviously, the US and Australian version should be avoided, although if the croissants are butter croissants (most are) and don't have a sugar glaze or a chocolate filling then they will, of course, be fine. If you want to spice it up a little, you could always do what those devil-may-care Europeans do and have a boiled egg.

Hot breakfasts

If you've got time, it's hard to go past the luxury of a hot breakfast. You can have eggs any way you like them (my favourite is pan-fried in butter) and pretty much any kind of meat (see the chart on page 126 for the best choices). If you have a hankering for bacon, then trim it to remove most of the grain-fed polyunsaturated fat or just don't have it that often. If meat isn't your thing, pan-fried mushrooms or tomatoes or some fresh avocado (don't have loads, though, a whole avocado has more than 4 grams of polyunsaturated fat) are good choices. I especially like sprinkling some salt in the frying pan, slicing a tomato in half and placing it cut sides down in the layer of salt. It gives a great salty crust to your cooked tomato. Did I mention that you don't need to worry about salt once you get rid of fructose (see page 32)? The amount of salt you eat should really be determined by just one thing – how much you like salt. If you're feeling really adventurous (or trying to impress someone), you could make a hollandaise or homemade tomato sauce instead (see the recipes in *Toxic Oil* for the hollandaise and Chapter 10 for the tomato sauce). If you like a hash brown with your fry-up, see Chapter 6 for pointers, but DIY will allow you to have as many as you like (see the recipe in *Toxic Oil*).

If you plan to do a fry-up every morning, veer towards free-range organic bacon, sausages, steak or lamb chops rather than ordinary bacon. Leave the bacon for a treat once or twice a week, to minimise exposure to seed oils. Have two eggs if you like (more than two eggs plus the bacon and you'll be consuming too much omega-6); they'll fill you up and provide you with just about every vitamin and mineral you need.

Shop-bought pancake mixes all have way too much sugar for real-food eaters. This doesn't mean you've eaten your last pancake; there's a sugar- and seed-oil-free recipe for them in Chapter 10. Our twins love these (especially the chocolate version) as a Sunday-morning treat. They serve them with some cream they whip themselves (don't let them do that in front of the telly – one morning we got butter instead of whipped cream), along with chopped-up bananas and frozen raspberries.

Savoury fritters (bubble-and-squeak) make a quick and filling hot breakfast that also has the advantage of using up leftovers. At first I resisted the idea because I thought it would be too much fuss and bother, but fritters are really quite easy. I can now whip up a batch in less time than it takes to cook toast, and they're absolutely delicious. I've included my savoury fritters recipe in *Toxic Oil*, but I can tell you what it is off the top of my head. Mix

300 grams of flour, 330 millilitres of milk and three large eggs in a bowl. Throw in chopped-up leftovers. Spoon into hot frying pan if your pan is non-stick. If it's not, pop in a little fat first. If you want them extra fluffy, use plain yoghurt instead of the milk. I promise you they're scrumptious.

THINGS TO HAVE FOR BREAKFAST AT HOME

- Unflavoured rolled oats (porridge) with full-cream milk
- Weet-Bix, Vita Brits or shredded wheat (unflavoured)
- Sugar-free muesli
- Toast with butter, Vegemite, cream cheese, peanut butter or avocado
- Boiled eggs (with toast soldiers, if you like) or omelette (especially good if you need to avoid flour)
- Eggs and bacon, sausages or steak, homemade hash brown, mushrooms or tomato (or the lot)
- Dextrose pancakes with berries and full-fat cream
- Savoury fritters

Drinks

Obviously, any drink that tastes sweet should be off the menu. There's only one real exception to this and it's one you might not expect. Lucozade Original is sweetened with glucose only. There isn't a drop of fructose in it. Our lot love it as a special treat every now and then. Be careful, though, as only the 'Original' flavour is sweetened with glucose. All the other varieties of Lucozade are sweetened with sugar or high-intensity sweeteners (mostly on the 'Your call' list; see page 117). This means that besides Lucozade, you're pretty much left with milk, water, tea and coffee.

The only place you're likely to encounter seed oil in a drink is in drinkable cereal products such as Sanitarium's Up&Go range: each 350-millilitre pack contains 2.5 grams of polyunsaturated fat and 26.6 grams (6.5 teaspoons) of sugar. For your interest, here's the ingredients list for Sanitarium Up&Go (Choc Ice flavour):

> filtered water, skim milk powder, cane sugar, wheat maltodextrin, soy protein, vegetable oils (sunflower, canola), hi-maize™ starch, corn syrup solids, inulin, fructose, cocoa (0.5%), cereals (oat flour, barley beta glucan), minerals (calcium, phosphorus), food acid (332), flavour, vegetable gums (460, 466, 407), vitamins (C, A, niacin, B12, B2, B6, B1, folate), salt.

'Food' like this must be avoided completely. If you don't have time to eat breakfast out of a bowl, might it be time to consider getting up twenty minutes earlier.

Personally, I like nothing better than a nice big glass of ice-cold, full-cream milk with my sausage and egg for breakfast. If you've been drinking low-fat milk your whole life and can't stomach the idea of full-fat, I'd advise you to try (given the research on the damage low-fat products could be doing to your LDL cholesterol count; see page 35), or else switch to water with your breakfast. (If you have milk in your tea or coffee, the amount is so small that it doesn't much matter whether you use full-fat or low-fat. If you make your coffee only with milk, you probably need to consider switching to full-fat milk or develop a taste for espresso shots.)

Lunch and dinner

You might eat your lunch at dinnertime or your dinner at lunchtime, so I've lumped these two meals together.

Sandwiches

If you know how the bread was made, sandwiches are a great option. The obvious traps for real-food eaters are in the spread and the condiments. If you're supplying the materials and the labour from your newly fake-food cleansed home then there's obviously nothing to fear. If, however, you're relying on the local sandwich shop, then you should make some requests. Ask them to use butter instead of margarine (and if they don't have butter then perhaps it's time to find a new sandwich shop). Ask them not to use mayonnaise. There's almost no chance that it's made without seed oils (if you want mayo at home there's a recipe in Chapter 10). And lastly, ask them not to add any sauces except mustard or gravy. Mustards are fine and gravy should be fine unless it tastes sweet.

As to the fillings, fresh anything will be good but avoid fried fillings (like chicken parma) or 'meats' (like rissoles) of uncertain heritage (probably not bad advice even if you aren't eating real food). After you've won their pesky customer of the year award you should be reasonably sure that your lunch is low in seed oils and sugar.

Salads

The best thing to put on a salad is air. The second best thing is your homemade dressing (mix a little olive oil with wholegrain or Dijon mustard and/or lime or lemon juice or vinegar, then throw in some herbs for taste). If you want to buy a made-up dressing, exercise extreme caution. Most are based on seed oils and some also have significant amounts of sugar (especially the low-fat versions). I haven't found one with acceptable levels of seed oils or sugar yet, but you never know your luck in the big supermarket.

Cooked food

Since you've restocked your pantry and fridge, you can pretty much cook whatever you want for lunch or dinner. This is why it's important to make sure you have only sugar-free and seed-oil-free food in the house. Your kitchen becomes a haven, where you know that every available ingredient is safe. You can combine anything with anything, knowing that whatever you cook for yourself and those you love won't be hurting you or them. Any kind of meat with any kind of vegetable makes for a good meal. You can have pasta, potatoes or rice with anything and know that as long as you're careful about the sauces you cook with (or add at the table), anything goes. If you're going Asian, veer towards Indian rather than Thai, but even then, in the safe harbour of your kitchen all the ingredients will be good no matter what style you choose. And if you're going with generic curry, use curry powder rather than a prepared paste.

Dessert

You might be surprised to find this section in your meal plan. Once you stop eating sugar you'll find you can rarely be bothered with the work required to create a non-addictive dessert. But if you can conjure up the desire (or need to feed people who expect dessert – that is, sugar eaters), there are a bunch of useful recipes in *The Sweet Poison Quit Plan* and *The Sweet Poison Quit*

Plan Cookbook. They are based on full-sugar recipes that my wife Lizzie and, in the case of the cookbook, professional chef Peta Dent have tweaked and modified (sometimes significantly) to make them taste very similar to the full-sugar original. The recipes in Chapter 10 include a few desserts we tend to make frequently. If a dessert you love isn't in any of these three books, pay close attention to the proportions of dextrose in something similar and you'll be able to modify your favourite recipe.

One thing you'll discover after you get through sugar withdrawal is that sweets in general lose much of their appeal. Lizzie can bake a chocolate cake in a house full of kids and have it last a week. It's not because it tastes bad, it's just not addictive. Once food isn't addictive, it's balanced fairly against other alternatives and, bizarre as it might sound to a fake-food eater, chocolate cake isn't always the most interesting-tasting alternative. So why have recipes for desserts at all? Most people tell me they like having a few dextrose recipes around for birthday parties and for when sugar-addicted guests drop over, but that's about it. No one seems to be bothered making desserts to have on hand every night.

Feeding kids

Obviously this section is for people who have munchkins to feed, so if that's not you, feel free to skip ahead – although if you occasionally take a packed lunch for yourself there might be a useful pointer or two.

You will by now have a completely seed-oil- and sugar-free home. And believe it or not, kids won't starve themselves to prove a point. If the only thing you have to drink comes from a tap or a cow, they'll choose one or the other. If the only snack you have is some lovely homemade biscuits, then guess what – they'll hoover them up. Of course, this won't stop them pigging out at parties or swapping lunches at school, but you will have controlled a significant majority of what goes in their mouth, and in so doing will probably have altered their palate (without them even realising you were doing it).

If you also explain why you're doing what you're doing and consistently apply it to yourself, they'll eventually see the benefits. They'll find they're sick less than their mates (sugar and seed oils depress the immune system). They'll find their moods are more even and life in general is easier to deal with. They even might find that many of the health problems that afflict their friends (such as acne and PCOS) pass them by. But none of that will help them overnight, so it's best to have some ground rules you can all play by. Here are my suggestions – based on running six kids through the highly successful 'Get the Gillespie Kids to Eat Real Food (most of the time) Program'.

USEFUL RULES TO HELP YOUR CHILDREN EAT REAL FOOD

Make sure that when you implement one of these rules, you explain why. Kids do understand that food can help and harm them, and as long as you're consistent and apply the same rules to yourself, they'll (eventually) toe the line.

1. **A sugar- and seed-oil-free home:** This must be an uncompromising and unchanging reality. If the only choice in the pantry is Dad's homemade olive oil bruschetta, then guess what's for afternoon tea.

---

2. **A sugar- and seed-oil-free lunch-box:** I know it's not possible to prepare food every day, but if you plan ahead you can come up with a freezer-load of things you can easily and quickly throw in a lunch-box. Lizzie will often bake a cake or biscuits on weekends, cling wrap them and freeze them ready for quick lunch-box assembly.

3. **Don't ban the tuckshop:** Kids like the tuckshop (no matter how appalling the food often is). See my rules for the tuckshop below.

4. **Keep an open mind:** Kids are always discovering new treats at the lunchtime-playground food exchange. If one of your kids suggests something new, take a good look at the ingredients – you never know, it may just be seed-oil- and sugar-free (or at least get through the fat and sugar rules on pages 141 and 143).

5. **Don't reward children with junk food:** A Macca's run or a chocolate bar at the supermarket is not a demonstration of love. Keeping them safe from the real damage those foods can do is. If your kids deserve a reward, take them to the movies or do something else with them. Don't fill them with stuff that seriously endangers their wellbeing.

6. **Prepare your kids for parties:** Kids go to parties. And you can be absolutely certain that they won't be chewing on carrot sticks and celery. You can't stop them eating their fill of sugar and seed oil just like their mates. But you can tell them why they shouldn't overdo it. And guess what, they often listen. Over time, kids develop a sense of responsibility for their own health and they often dial down the binge. But even if they don't, as long as you keep the rest of their life

as sugar- and seed-oil-free as possible, they're unlikely to do themselves real harm.

7. **Give a teenager options:** There's only one thing that matters more to a teenager than how they look, and that's what everyone else thinks of them. If all their friends are hanging out at Macca's then that's where they'll be too. The best thing you can do for them in that situation is tell them the best choices they can make from a bad lot. Direct them to the diet drinks, tell them to order their burger without sauce, and suggest they avoid the fries. In short, provide them with a strategy that doesn't mark them out as a weirdo but still preserves their health (as best you can).

8. **Only eat fried food at home:** Most commercial takeaway food is fried in seed oils. If you want your kids to be able to enjoy fried food occasionally, it's best to cook it at home in healthy traditional fats like lard or olive oil.

I'm no professional child wrangler, but it seems to me that you've got to give kids a little room to adjust. Don't expect them to elect you parent of the month when you introduce these rules, but remember that eventually they'll adjust to the reality that sugar and seed oils are no longer part of your (or their) lives. And the older they get, the more they'll appreciate why.

All that being said, you can do some things to dramatically reduce the sugar and seed oil in children's lives without making them feel deprived.

Breakfast for kids

Here's what our six kids had for breakfast this morning.

A BREAKFAST FOR SIX (KIDS)

Child 1 (male, eighteen): two fried eggs and two reheated beef sausages

Child 2 (male, seventeen): two fried eggs, two sausages, three pieces of Vegemite toast

Child 3 (female, fifteen): one piece of toast with rice malt syrup and one piece of Vegemite toast

Child 4 (male, fourteen): one fried egg and one sausage (can you tell we had some sausages we needed to offload?)

Child 5 (female, eleven): two pieces of sourdough toast with avocado

Child 6 (female, eleven): two pieces of buttered toast and a banana

They all had a glass of full-cream milk to wash it down.

The toast is made using homemade bread from the recipes in Chapter 10, and is spread with butter, not margarine. Avocado is a great thing to spread on a piece of toast, but a medium-sized (240-gram) avocado will have about 4.3 grams of polyunsaturated fat, so it's a good idea to keep the serving to about a quarter of a fruit (providing about 1 gram of polyunsaturated fat) in any one sitting. Vegemite is a great alternative that kids tend to like (as long as they've been raised on it). Whenever anyone can be bothered to cook, it will be middle rashers of bacon or sausages, egg, tomato and maybe some mushrooms, or just a boiled egg with toast soldiers for those who aren't so keen on fry-ups.

School lunches

There are really no processed-food options for lunch-boxes. Muesli and snack bars are loaded with sugar, and you won't be dropping in any boxes of sultanas or juice. It's mostly DIY with school lunches, unfortunately.

Unflavoured popcorn is a great sugar-free morning tea that stays edible in a schoolbag. Either buy the corn kernels yourself, pop them in a saucepan (with a bit of olive oil) and put them in zip-lock baggies, or just buy unflavoured popped corn (just be careful to check what oil was used to pop the corn – it will say it in the ingredients list). Microwave popcorn is pre-cooked in a palm- and seed-oil blend, so it's not a great choice. One hundred grams contains around 3.4 grams of polyunsaturated fat versus 2 grams for home-popped corn. Popcorn is light, though, so the average kid is probably only eating 25–40 grams in a serving, which means that if time isn't on your side, you can get away with microwave popcorn without worrying too much about its seed-oil content.

Of course, fresh fruit is an option. And while you should veer towards fruits that are low in fructose and high in fibre (such as berries or kiwifruit), don't worry too much about it if this is the only fruit they'll be having in the average day.

Of course, you can always throw a small bag of plain salted crisps into the lunch-box. They contain no sugar and the high-oleic sunflower oil (see Chapter 6) used is even lower in polyunsaturated fat than olive oil.

If you're parent of the year, you'll be reaching into the freezer and pulling out a slice of homemade cake, a muffin or a biscuit you whipped up on the weekend using dextrose instead of sugar.

SOME IDEAS FOR 'LITTLE LUNCH/PLAYLUNCH/RECESS'

- Berries or any one piece of whole fruit
- Homemade popcorn
- Unflavoured cracker biscuits
- Crisps
- Homemade dextrose biscuits or cakes (from *The Sweet Poison Quit Plan* or *The Sweet Poison Quit Plan Cookbook*)

For lunch, sandwiches or rolls are a good way to go. One of the current favourites at our place is the roast beef roll: leftover roast beef, whacked on an olive-oil-based hamburger roll (that we convinced our local Bakers Delight to make for us) with homemade olive-oil mayo and lettuce – yum.

Another lunchtime treat that's become popular with our kids is 'fish and chips': a small tin of canned tuna (or the fish of their choice) and a small bag of plain potato crisps (avoid flavoured crisps). Just remember to check the canned tuna ingredients. Tuna in spring water is the best choice. Even if a tin proclaims that it is canned in olive oil, it's probably really just seed oil that's had a little olive oil added so they can make that claim.

Drinks are easy: fill drink bottles with water and freeze them. If children don't want water, they're not thirsty. The temperature is far more important than the taste to a hot and bothered schoolkid.

Yoghurt and yoghurt-like snacks (often called 'dairy treats' or 'dairy snacks') aren't an option for the lunch-box or for home. They're invariably very high in sugar (otherwise most kids wouldn't touch them, as yoghurt is intrinsically sour). Unfortunately, there's no low-sugar option available in this type of food unless you want to stray into artificial sweeteners or serve plain yoghurt. The same thing applies to stewed-fruit snacks; they're usually served in a fruit syrup and have a significant proportion of the fibre removed because they're peeled. If fruit is what your children want, give them fresh fruit or frozen berries. Once your kids lose the taste for sugar, they'll find Greek yoghurt quite appealing, especially if you stir through some berries, some dextrose and a bit of vanilla essence.

Beware, though, that as your children's appetite control returns to normal, letting them fill up with yoghurt, crisps, popcorn or dextrose treats at afternoon tea will mean they don't feel much like eating dinner (no matter how fabulous a cook you are).

The tuckshop

Unfortunately, rocketing childhood obesity rates have meant that school tuckshops have become the frontline in the war on unhealthy eating. Meat pies and sausage rolls have been banned. Soft drinks have been replaced with fruit juices and flavoured milks. Sweets have been replaced with dried fruit, butter with margarine and all frying (if any) is done in 'vegetable oil'. In other words, they've systematically turned the average tuckshop into a place you'd have to pay most children to eat and at the same time managed to make all the food lethal. The result is that fewer low-sugar options are available in the 'healthy' tuckshop than there were in the bad old days, and very few options aren't filled to the brim with seed oils. If the tuckshop is your only option for a meal, here are a few guidelines.

RULES FOR TUCKSHOPS

- Don't purchase anything fried.
- Don't use any sauces or dressings and if one is included ask for it to be made without.
- If the sandwiches, wraps or burgers don't contain anything fried or sauce/dressing, they're fine, but ask that they not be spread with margarine.
- If they have sausage rolls, sausages in bread or pies available, they're a good choice (without the sauce).
- Drink only unflavoured full-fat milk or water (sparkling is fine too).
- Don't purchase fruit-like products except actual whole fruit.
- Skip the yoghurt unless it's the plain, unsweetened variety.

Party food

Kids like treats as much as the rest of us. The recipes in *The Sweet Poison Quit Plan* and *The Sweet Poison Quit Plan Cookook* focus especially on sweet treats. Birthday cakes, ice-creams, cupcakes and icing are necessary for birthday parties and other special occasions. But in a shop they're impossible to find without vast amounts of sugar and – if there's any crispy component – large amounts of seed oil, just for good measure.

10
RECIPES

This isn't a recipe book. No chefs, food stylists, nutritionists or photographers were involved in its construction. But if you're going to Eat Real Food, you're going to need some basic recipes. Sure, I could introduce you to the wonders of Google and the internet, but Lizzie and I have been living this for the last decade, so we've learnt a few things along the way. This section is for us to provide you with the recipes we've found we just can't live without. They're not flash. They don't use expensive or difficult-to-find ingredients. You won't be asked to buy a single coconut product or manhandle a single acai berry. These recipes are for common garden-variety foods you would have to have made yourself before supermarkets were invented. All the recipes are simple, quick enough to make on a daily basis if you want to, and – best of all – made from real food. Just for fun, next to the ingredients for each recipe, I've listed the ingredients of a typical example of a processed food of that type, along with a cost comparison.

If you look closely, you'll notice another theme that ties these recipes together. We now make a lot of food that we used to buy. The only way that's sustainable in a busy family is if we can make significant shortcuts. Over the years, Lizzie has developed ways to create an array of common foods from the same base recipe and a very limited set of ingredients. So you'll see, for example, that the bread and bread-like recipes are almost all based on just one recipe. If you have flour, yeast and oil to hand, you can make any of the recipes or all of them. The same goes for the custard recipe, which is microscopically adjusted to become a baked custard, a crème brûlée or even an ice-cream. These recipes are designed to be functional for constant use in busy households. You'll find everything you need at the local shop and you'll be able to buy all of it in bulk because you know the recipes are all designed to use similar ingredients. Welcome to *The Little House on the Prairie*.

Some ground rules

Before you tie on your apron, here are a few things you should know about some of the ingredients we use:

- **Dextrose** is dextrose monohydrate. You should be able to buy it in 1-kilogram bags from the home-brew section of your local supermarket (for about $3). If it's not available, there are plenty of specialist home-brew shops that can supply it in bulk. It's the glucose half of sugar, which means it's sugar that's effectively had the dangerous fructose half deleted. Dextrose looks like caster sugar but is nowhere near as sweet, although the recipes that use it have been carefully chosen so that most people (even those who still eat sugar) won't be able to tell the difference (usually because the sugar-based version of the recipe isn't that sweet either).

- Dextrose-based foods (especially cakes and biscuits) tend not to last as long as sugar-based equivalents (sugar is a preservative), so keep them in the fridge or freezer until you plan to eat them.
- When a recipe says **cream,** we use thickened cream. This doesn't necessarily mean that ordinary cream won't work just as well, but we know the recipe works well with thickened cream.
- We use extra-large (at least 59-gram) **eggs.** We don't know how well most of these recipes work with smaller eggs, so you could be throwing the dice if that's all you've got.
- When a recipe says **butter,** we use unsalted butter. Dextrose is a very weak sweetener and salted butter can overpower it, but if it's not a sweet recipe then it doesn't matter if you used salted butter. You can spend a lot on flash butter but we just buy the home-brand stuff in bulk.
- When a recipe calls for **vanilla essence,** we sometimes don't specify a quantity because how much you use depends on your personal taste. Generally, half to one teaspoon (maximum) gives a good result. When we do suggest a quantity, take it as just that, a suggestion.

- When a recipe calls for **salt**, once again it's about personal taste. Put in as much or as little as you like. I only specify an amount so I can add a number for the cost.

- All the **prices** I've used are full retail prices for the ingredients and their comparative products as at the end of 2014. You'll be able to buy many of the ingredients at much lower prices (especially the vegetables), so I suggest you do as Lizzie and I do, and keep an eye on the specials. Since you now Eat Real Food made from real ingredients, the price of those ingredients can have a dramatic impact on the amount you pay for food overall. And even though most of the end products you make are less than half the cost of their processed cousins even at full price, if you're a little bit mindful of ingredient prices you can do even better.

Homemade bread

There's nothing like the smell of freshly baked bread and there's nothing like the taste of the hot crusty end piece smeared with butter. But, if you do it wrong, bread-making can take up an awful lot of time and completely put you off the process. The recipes that follow have been refined over many years of use to deliver hot bread with minimum effort and maximum yum. We don't use a bread machine, but if you did it would get even easier. Lizzie tends to make a loaf of bread by hand in the afternoon – it takes her just minutes of hands-on effort – and we eat most of it as toast over the following two mornings. This, by the way, is significantly less bread than we used to eat when we could just buy it four loaves at a time from the supermarket (hey, we have teenage boys!). A combination of the extra effort to make it and the bread being less more-ish (it has no sugar) has cut back our consumption significantly.

Yeasted bread

In the spirit of trying to have just a few good recipes that can be put to multiple uses, this one isn't only perfect for bread, it's also an excellent pizza-base recipe, and makes fabulous cheese and bacon rolls, not to mention breadcrumbs, of course. We've included all these variations from this one simple recipe in the following pages.

Lizzie first used this recipe for pizza dough but noticed how easy it was to knead (because it's a wetter mix than normal bread recipes), and how well it rose when left to prove. Lizzie uses one of those marble breadboards to knead it on (so she doesn't need any extra flour for dusting). She decided to try baking it as a loaf one week, and hasn't looked back. And if there are any bits left over, it also makes great breadcrumbs. The use of semolina in the last knead before shaping your loaf helps create a crisper crust but isn't really necessary.

If supermarket white is what you're after then this loaf will disappoint. It's similar fresh, but crumblier and less springy when cold. It still makes terrific toast, though, and the bread eaters in our family certainly have no complaints. But the very best thing about it (besides the price) is you can be absolutely certain that it contains not one added gram of seed oils or sugar.

Pro-Tip: Make sure the water is lukewarm – too hot and it will kill the yeast, too cold and the yeast won't activate.

Makes 1 loaf (10 × 21 cm)

INGREDIENTS

4½ cups plain flour, plus extra for dusting

2 generous teaspoons (1 sachet) dried yeast

1 teaspoon salt

1½ cups lukewarm water

¼ cup extra virgin olive oil

¼ cup semolina (optional)

METHOD

1. Preheat oven to 200°C. Grease and flour a 10 × 21 cm loaf tin.
2. In a bowl, mix together flour, yeast and salt.
3. Make a well in the dry ingredients and pour in warm water and olive oil. Mix to bring dough together. Because this is quite a wet mix to begin with, Lizzie kneads it in the bowl until it is less sticky and can be kneaded on the board (without added flour).
4. Turn dough onto a smooth, clean, dry surface and form it into a ball. Now, using the heel of your hand, push the centre of the ball of dough down and away from you. Then bring the far edge of the dough up and back towards you, and press it into the middle of the ball again until the dough is soft and smooth (approximately 8 minutes). You can use the dough hook on your mixer instead if you prefer. You'll know when it's done because it is smooth and a nudge from your finger will bounce back.
5. When you're happy with the consistency, place the ball of dough in a buttered (or olive-oiled) bowl, cover with cling wrap and leave in a warm place to prove for an hour or until it has doubled in size.
6. Once dough has doubled in size, sprinkle some flour or the semolina (if you have it) mixed in with the flour on your kneading surface. Then take the dough out of the bowl, put it on the lightly floured surface, and knead until smooth.
7. Shape into a loaf, cut three grooves diagonally across the top of the loaf and gently place in the tin.

8. Place tin in a warm, draught-free spot (over the top of the oven is a good place) until loaf has doubled in size (this should take about 30 minutes).
9. Place in oven (be aware that the loaf may rise further, so don't crowd it with the shelves above) and bake for about 30 minutes or until loaf is crusty and sounds hollow when tapped.
10. (Optional: At about the 20-minute mark, spritz it with a little water while in the oven to give the crust a bit of a glaze.)
11. Turn loaf out of tin and cool on a wire rack before cutting.

COSTINGS

Ingredients	Weight/ Volume	Cost	Processed alternative	Weight	Cost
4½ cups plain flour	600 g	$0.45	Coles Sliced White: Wheat flour, water, fibre (5%) (soy), yeast, vinegar, canola oil, iodised salt, wheat gluten, soy flour, vegetable emulsifiers (471, 481), mineral salt (calcium carbonate), vitamins (vitamin E, niacin, thiamine, vitamin B6, folic acid), minerals (iron, zinc)	700 g	$2.30
2 generous teaspoons (1 sachet) dried yeast	7 g	$0.12			
1 teaspoon salt	5.7 g	$0.01			
1½ cups lukewarm water	325 ml	$0.00			
¼ cup extra virgin olive oil	62.5 ml	$0.44			
¼ cup semolina (optional)	44 g	$0.12			
Final loaf	940 g	$1.14		700 g	$2.30

Cheese and bacon bread rolls or pull-aparts

Our kids love cheese and bacon rolls, especially when they're warm and fresh from the oven. You can, of course, make them with any topping you like. The following recipe is exactly the same as the bread recipe above for the first six steps of the method. Only the last few steps of the method change, but I've included the whole thing again for ease of reference.

Makes 8 large or 16 small rolls or one large pull-apart

INGREDIENTS

4½ cups plain flour, plus extra for dusting

2 generous teaspoons (1 sachet) dried yeast

1 teaspoon salt

1½ cups lukewarm water

¼ cup extra virgin olive oil

¼ cup semolina (optional)

200 g bacon, diced

250 g cheese, grated

METHOD

1. Preheat oven to 200°C. Grease a baking tray or line it with baking paper.
2. In a bowl, mix together flour, yeast and salt.
3. Make a well in the dry ingredients and pour in warm water and olive oil. Mix to bring dough together. Because this is quite a wet mix to begin with, Lizzie kneads it in the bowl until it is less sticky and can be kneaded on the board (without added flour).
4. Turn dough onto a smooth, clean, dry surface and form it into a ball. Now, using the heel of your hand, push the centre of the ball of dough down and away from you. Then bring the far edge of the dough up and back towards you, and press it into the middle of the ball again until the dough is soft and smooth (approximately 8 minutes). You can use the dough hook on your mixer instead if you prefer. You'll know when it's done because it is smooth and a nudge from your finger will bounce back.
5. When you're happy with the consistency, place the ball of dough in a buttered (or olive-oiled) bowl, cover with cling wrap and leave in a warm place to prove for an hour or until it has doubled in size.

6. Once dough has doubled in size, sprinkle some flour or the semolina (if you have it) mixed in with the flour on your kneading surface. Then take the dough out of the bowl, put it on the lightly floured surface, and knead until smooth.
7. Split the dough into 8 (or 16) lumps, round them up in your hands and place on the prepared baking tray.
8. Push your favourite grated cheese into the top (or olives or your favourite herbs – do whatever you like, really – treat it as an adventure). Then push diced raw bacon into the tops (to taste in terms of quantity).
9. Alternatively, you could divide the dough into three long tubes, plait them and then add the bacon and cheese to create a bacon and cheese pull-apart.
10. Set aside somewhere warm to rise for about 30 minutes.
11. Place in oven (be aware that the bread may rise further so don't crowd it with the shelves above) and bake for about 30 minutes (of course smaller rolls will take less time to cook) or until bread is crusty and sounds hollow when tapped.
12. (Optional: At about the 20-minute mark, spritz it with a little water while in the oven to give the crust a bit of a glaze.)
13. Cool on a wire rack before serving.

COSTINGS

Ingredients	Weight/Volume	Cost	Processed alternative	Weight	Cost
4½ cups plain flour	600 g	$0.45	Coles Cheese and Bacon Rolls (4 packs of 4 [350 g]): Wheat flour, cheese (14%) (milk, salt, cultures, rennet, preservative [235]), bacon (14%) (pork, salt, dextrose, sugar, mineral salts [450, 451, 452], water, antioxidant [316], preservative [250]), water, yeast, wheat gluten, vegetable oil (canola, palm), iodised salt, soy flour, sugar, vitamins (thiamine, folic acid)	1400 g	$17.60
2 generous teaspoons (1 sachet) dried yeast	7 g	$0.12			
1 teaspoon salt	5.7 g	$0.01			
1½ cups lukewarm water	325 ml	$0.00			
¼ cup extra virgin olive oil	62.5 ml	$0.44			
¼ cup semolina (optional)	44 g	$0.25			
200 g diced bacon	200 g	$3.47			
250 g cheese	250 g	$4.40			
Final bread	1390 g	$9.14		1400 g	$17.60

Pizza dough

The ingredients and amounts are exactly the same as for the yeasted bread but I've reproduced them here for ease of reference.

Makes 10 small thin and crispy pizza bases

INGREDIENTS

4½ cups plain flour, plus extra for dusting

2 generous teaspoons (1 sachet) dried yeast

1 teaspoon salt

1½ cups lukewarm water

¼ cup extra virgin olive oil

¼ cup semolina (optional)

METHOD

1. In a bowl, mix together flour, yeast and salt.
2. Make a well in the dry ingredients and pour in warm water and olive oil. Mix to bring dough together.
3. Turn mixture onto a floured surface and knead until a smooth, elastic dough forms (approximately 8 minutes).
4. When you're happy with the consistency, place ball of dough in a buttered (or olive-oiled) bowl, cover with cling wrap and leave in a warm place for 30 minutes, if there's time.
5. Preheat oven to 210°C.
6. Divide dough evenly into the number of pizzas you plan to make.
7. Roll out on bench sprinkled with mixture of semolina and flour and add toppings (whatever you like). Then place the pizzas in the preheated oven for 15 minutes or until they look cooked (which usually means the cheese is melted and beginning to brown).
8. You will, of course, need a sauce for your pizza base. You'll find a recipe for that on page 266.

COSTINGS

Ingredients	Weight/ Volume	Cost	Processed alternative	Weight	Cost
4½ cups plain flour	600 g	$0.45	Mission Plain Pizza Bases (5 double packs of 200 g): Wheat flour (65%) (thiamine, folic acid), water, vegetable shortening (antioxidant [320]), bread improver (wheat flour, thickener [412], barley malt extract, acidity regulators [339, 341, 340], wheat malt flour, emulsifier [472e], whey powder, antioxidant [300]), wheat sourdough, sugar, yeast, iodised salt, food acid (297), bread improver (barley malt extract, pregelatinised wholemeal rye flour, acidity regulator [270]), baking powder (mineral salts [500, 450, 341]), preservative (282)	1 kg	$19.95
2 generous teaspoons (1 sachet) dried yeast	7 g	$0.12			
1 teaspoon salt	5.7 g	$0.01			
1½ cups lukewarm water	325 ml	$0.00			
¼ cup extra virgin olive oil	62.5 ml	$0.44			
¼ cup semolina (optional)	44 g	$0.25			
Final bases	940 g	$1.27		1 kg	$19.95

Garlic bread

If you're having pizza, then garlic bread is likely to be on the menu too. Here's a quick and easy way to produce perfect buttered garlic bread without the hassle of doing it (all) yourself. If garlic isn't your thing, then just substitute herbs such as rosemary and thyme to turn this into a toasted herb bread instead.

INGREDIENTS
1 small Coles Baked White Sourdough Baguette*
100 g butter, softened
1 large clove (or 2 small cloves) garlic

METHOD
1. Preheat oven to 180°C.
2. Make twenty diagonal slices in the baguette using a serrated bread knife – don't cut all the way through.
3. Crush the garlic into the butter and mix with a spoon.
4. Using a butter knife, distribute the butter evenly between your twenty cuts.
5. Wrap the whole loaf in aluminium foil and heat in oven for 10–15 minutes or until butter is melted and bread is warm.
6. Alternatively, you can freeze the loaf (in its foil) then heat it later. This allows you to be strategic about when you buy the bread, because it can often be on special (the prices below are full prices).

COSTINGS

Ingredients	Weight/ Volume	Cost	Processed alternative	Weight	Cost
1 small Coles Baked White Sourdough Baguette*	300 g	$3.00	La Famiglia Garlic Bread (2 nine slice packs) Bread: (70%) [Wheat Flour (Vitamins (Thiamin, Folic Acid)), Water, Yeast, Iodised Salt, Wheat Gluten, Vegetable Oil, Soy Flour, Emulsifiers (481, 471), Mineral Salt (Calcium Carbonate), Preservative (282)]. Spread: (30%) [Margarine, Vegetable Oil, Water, Salt, Milk Solids, Emulsifiers (471, Soyabean Lecithin), Flavour, Antioxidant (320), Colour (160a)), Vegetable Oil, Garlic Oil (<1%), Dried Parsley (<1%)]. NOTE: Emulsifiers 471 and 481 are of Vegetable Origin and Extraction.	540 g	$11.34
100 g softened butter	100 g	$0.59			
1 large clove (or 2 small cloves) garlic	10 g	$0.12			
Final bread	410 g	$3.71		540 g	$11.34

*   Ingredients for the Coles Sourdough: wheat flour, water, sourdough (water, wheat flour, rye flour), iodised salt, soy flour, malt powder, wheat bran, yeast, vitamins (thiamine, folic acid). You could, of course, just make your own using half the bread recipe above and shaping it into a French stick before baking.

Breadcrumbs

In our place, there are often leftover end bits of bread – mostly because children seem to get all random when it comes to wielding a bread knife. We keep those hardened stale ends (in a plastic container in the fridge) and every few weeks shove them into a food processor. A few seconds later, we have perfect breadcrumbs. Obviously, the ingredients and method are exactly the same as for making bread (if you're even inspired to make perfectly good bread just to turn it into crumbs) but for the sake of comparison, here's that costings table. (See also 'Something to do with breadcrumbs' on page 255.)

COSTINGS

Ingredients	Weight/Volume	Cost	Processed alternative	Weight	Cost
4½ cups plain flour	600 g	$0.45	Coles Smart Buy Breadcrumbs (2 packs of 500 g): Wheat flour, wholemeal wheat flour, malted wheat flour, rye flour, malted barley flour, rye meal, soy flour, mixed grains (kibbled rye, kibbled wheat, wheat bran, buckwheat, kibbled sorghum, triticale, kibbled barley, kibbled purple wheat, kibbled corn, malted wheat flake, oat bran, millet, rolled oats, maize semolina), mixed seeds (linseed, sunflower seeds, pumpkin seeds, flaxseed, sesame seeds, poppy seeds), yeast, cereal fibre (maize, oat), wheat gluten, iodised salt, canola oil, kibbled soy, kibbled maize, quinoa, wheat semolina, soy fibre, vinegar, sugar, molasses, vegetable gum (412, 414), cultured wheat flour, wheat germ, wheat starch, emulsifiers (481 [vegetable], 471 [vegetable], 472e [vegetable]), mineral salt (calcium carbonate), skim milk powder, vitamins (folic acid, thiamine, niacin, vitamin E, vitamin B6), minerals (iron, zinc)	1 kg	$3.40
2 generous teaspoons (1 sachet) dried yeast	7 g	$0.12			
1 teaspoon salt	5.7 g	$0.01			
1½ cups lukewarm water	325 ml	$0.00			
¼ cup extra virgin olive oil	62.5 ml	$0.44			
¼ cup semolina (optional)	44 g	$0.25			
Final breadcrumbs	940 g	$1.27		1 kg	$3.40

Sourdough bread

Sourdough bread should perfectly fit the criteria of no sugar and no seed oils. And while most commercial sourdough is sugar-free, most supermarket sourdough loaves are now made with canola oil. At Coles, only the 'Rustic' sourdough is free from seed oils, and Woolies doesn't seem to have any options without seed oils. Most of our kids prefer the white bread (recipe above) toasted for breakfast. But there is one (plus Lizzie and I) who really enjoys the slight tang of a traditional sourdough with some yummy mashed avocado, salt and pepper. This fantastic recipe takes less than five minutes of prep and involves no kneading (or any other messing about).

Most sourdough recipes call for kneading, but that was a messy procedure with this very sticky wet dough, so one morning I didn't bother and it seemed to have no effect on the end product. That little shortcut has made this recipe cosmically simple. But if you don't have someone getting up early to put your bread in the oven, just mix the ingredients after brekkie, leave the mix to stand all day and cook it in the evening. It's still scrumptiously fresh the next morning.

The starter

This might look like a lot of steps but they're simple steps and you only do this once. The trick to this recipe is having a 'starter' – a culture of a yeast-like substance that you feed with flour every few days or so. This is really just yoghurt bacteria that you're going to keep alive in a jar in your fridge. Our sourdough starter has been going strong for the past four years. We even take it on holidays with us. It just sits there in the corner of the fridge in its little jar, brewing up tomorrow's bread. Once your starter is established, you'll be removing some to make bread and replacing what you take with some flour and water so as to keep it going.

IMPORTANT: your starter mustn't be contaminated with any commercial yeasts because the stronger strains will take over. So always use a clean spoon to deal with your starter (removing, replenishing and mixing) in its container. When your starter is brand new (you've only made a few loaves), you might need to add some dried yeast to your bread dough (but not the starter) because the bacteria in the starter are not quite up to the job of getting a good rise out of your dough.

Pro-Tip: If you want to make a new starter (what a nice birthday present) just take a little of your old one out and put it in a new jar with water and flour.

plain flour
water
natural yoghurt (we use Greek)

Day 1: Find a jar to store the starter in. You need something that will protect the contents without being completely airtight. We use a large old glass Moccona coffee jar (with the pop-top plastic-based lid). You can use a bowl if you like, but it takes up a lot of space in the fridge. In the jar, mix together **50 grams flour, 50 ml water and 2 tablespoons yoghurt.** Put the lid on the jar (or cover the bowl with cling film) and leave somewhere warm (out of the fridge but not hot) overnight.

Day 2: Using a clean spoon, add **100 grams flour and 100 ml water**. Mix to combine, re-cover and re-place in its warm spot.

Day 3: Today you will be taking some starter out (and making bread with it if you want to) and putting some new flour and water in. Remove 200 grams from your starter to make your first loaf (see method below). At this stage, the starter will give your loaf sourdough flavour, but it's still weak, so you'll need some yeast to make bread – see below. If you don't want to make bread until you can do it without yeast, simply discard the 200 grams. Either way, replenish (once again with a clean spoon) with **100 grams flour and 100 ml water**. Mix to combine, re-cover and re-place in its warm spot.

Day 4: From now on, repeat the removal of 200 grams of starter each day (or every second day, you don't need to be too precise about it), either discarding or baking with it (with yeast at this stage), and replenishing with **100 grams flour and 100 ml water** before combining, re-covering and re-placing in its warm spot.

Days 10–15: At some point, you'll begin to notice that your starter becomes quite a bit more active (be patient – this may take a week or so longer in colder climates and/or winter). It will obviously bubble in the bottle. Due to that aeration, it will appear to almost double in size between refills. Once this is happening, your starter is established. You can now keep it in the fridge (to stop it growing too fast) and use it to bake sourdough without the need for yeast. Plan to 'feed' your starter twice a week (removing 200 grams and replenishing using a clean spoon with 100 grams flour and 100 ml water), or more frequently if you're baking more often. Sometimes it won't look like there's much starter left after you take your 200 grams out, but not to worry, once you have an established starter you can restart it with just a very small sample of the original. Even if all you have left is a dirty jar, that will be enough to get it going again.

Pro-Tip: Invest in a set of kitchen scales that allow you to zero the balance once you've put something on them (we got ours from the post office for $10). That way, it's very easy to add the 100 grams flour and 100 ml water by simply putting the starter on the scales, zeroing them and adding flour until they hit 100 grams, then zeroing them again and pouring in water until they hit 100 grams again – 100 ml water weighs 100 grams, so if you're using this method you can substitute the volume measurement for the same number of grams.

The sourdough loaf

Makes 1 loaf (10 × 21 cm)

INGREDIENTS
200 g sourdough starter (see above)
2½ cups plain flour, plus extra for dusting
275 ml water
pinch of fine-grained salt (optional)
¼ teaspoon dried yeast (if starter not yet established)

METHOD
1. In a large bowl, mix together starter, flour, water and salt (and yeast if starter isn't yet established). Cover with cling wrap and leave to stand in a warm place for at least 8 hours (12 if possible).
2. Preheat oven to 200°C, and grease and flour a 10 × 21 cm loaf tin. (Or if, like us, you're using a reinforced silicone tin, this doesn't need greasing or flouring.) If you're really old school, you could use a cast iron pot to get a nice round (cobb shaped) loaf.
3. Using a plastic kitchen scraper/spatula (the mix is sticky and elastic – easy to manipulate with a plastic scraper but impossible with anything else), pour the mix into the tin. Sit the tin on a metal oven tray and place in oven.
4. Bake for 45 minutes or until loaf is crusty and sounds hollow when tapped.
5. Turn loaf out of tin and cool on a wire rack for about 30 minutes (if you can stand waiting – I usually can't and so burn my fingers cutting off the crust for a 'preview'), before slicing and enjoying. It tastes great fresh but after a day or so, it's better toasted.

COSTINGS

Ingredients	Weight/ Volume	Cost	Processed alternative	Weight	Cost
200 g sourdough starter	200 g	$0.15	Schwob's White Sourdough: Wheat flour (folic acid), water, yeast, iodised salt, skim milk powder, shortening (animal fat, vegetable oil (antioxidant [307]), water, emulsifiers (471, 472e), salt, food acid (330), flavour, antioxidant [320]), liquid sour (1%) (rye flour, malt extract, acetic acid), soya flour, vinegar, bread improver (wheat flour, emulsifier [472e], flour treatment agent [ascorbic acid], enzymes)	800 g	$5.10
2½ cups plain flour	325 g	$0.24			
275 ml water	275 ml	$0.00			
Pinch of fine-grained salt	0 g	$0.00			
¼ teaspoon dried yeast (if starter not yet established)	0.7 g	$0.01			
Final loaf	620 g	$0.40		800 g	$5.10

Savoury

Meat pie

Most frozen pies are less than 25 per cent meat and contain vegetable oil. The amount of vegetable oil wouldn't normally be much of a concern because, using the fat rules on page 143, it looks like they're using old-fashioned cooking margarines (which are dominated by animal fats). But we prefer no added seed oils if we can manage it, and we also wanted to increase the meat content, so we set about making our own. Like many of the things I thought would be too much trouble to make on a regular basis, meat pies turned out to be so simple they're now a staple in the Gillespie household.

This recipe makes one large (25 cm) deep meat pie. It satisfies the eight of us (the equivalent of four adults and four kids) when served with vegetables for dinner. We've also made it into single-serve pies. We tend to make up a batch of filling and freeze it, then thaw and make the pie with puff (or homemade, see recipe) pastry just before we're going to eat it.

You can fandangle this recipe quite a bit by adding in mushrooms or onion with the meat at the start. We also often make this gluten-free (for a relative) by replacing the flour in the filling with a gluten-free alternative and make it as a shepherd's pie – in a baking dish with a mashed-potato top (instead of a pastry-encased pie).

Serves 8

INGREDIENTS

1 tablespoon extra virgin olive oil

1 kg casserole beef, untrimmed, diced

2 generous tablespoons Bonox (about one-third of a 230 g bottle)

3 heaped tablespoons plain flour

1 cup cold water, plus extra for cooking

2 sheets frozen butter puff pastry (or one batch of homemade
   pastry – see recipe)

METHOD

1. Heat oil in a large saucepan over medium heat.
2. Add beef and Bonox, moving them around a little to ensure the
   meat is browned but doesn't burn.
3. Meanwhile, in a separate bowl, gradually mix together flour
   and water, stirring until there are no lumps. Set aside. For the
   technically inclined this is called making a slurry.
4. Pour extra water into saucepan until meat is almost covered. Then
   add flour and water mix. Cover and bring to the boil. Allow to boil
   for 5 minutes, covered.
5. Uncover and simmer (stirring occasionally so meat doesn't catch
   on base of saucepan) for at least 2 hours or until meat has broken
   down and has a thick, gravy-like consistency. Remove from heat.
   If you don't want to use the filling straight away, freeze it in an
   airtight container.
6. When ready to assemble, defrost filling if frozen. Preheat oven to
   200°C. Grease a 25 cm pie tin.
7. Take the first sheet of puff pastry, place it in the pie dish and prick
   the bottom. (Store-bought puff pastry may be a bit smaller than
   your dish; roll it out a little, and cut and paste any overhang to
   where it's needed.)
8. Add filling on top of pastry. Wet your finger and run it round the
   pastry base edge then place second sheet of pastry over the top
   and press into edges of the pie to attach to base.
9. If you want to get fancy, use the pastry off-cuts to make little
   decorations for the top of the pie.
10. Bake for 30–45 minutes or until golden brown. Serve.

COSTINGS

Ingredients	Weight/ Volume	Cost	Processed alternative	Weight	Cost
1 tablespoon extra virgin olive oil	13.7 ml	$0.10	Sargents Aussie Angus Beef Family Pie (2 packs of 550 g): Water, Angus beef (28%), wheat flour, margarine (animal fat and vegetable oil, water, salt, emulsifier [471, 322 (soy)], milk solids, antioxidants [304, 306 (soy), 320], acidity regulator [330], flavour, colour [160a]), thickener (1422 [maize]), textured vegetable protein (soy), flavour (yeast extract, soy protein isolate, spice and spice extract, maltodextrin [wheat], lactose [milk]), salt, onion powder, dextrose, colours (150c, 160b, 160a), herbs and spices (wheat), pastry glaze (milk, wheat, thickener [464])	1100 g	$14.30
1 kg casserole beef	1 kg	$10.00			
2 generous tablespoons Bonox	75 g	$2.97			
3 heaped tablespoons plain flour	23.5 g	$0.01			
1 cup cold water, plus extra for cooking	250 ml	$0.00			
2 sheets frozen butter puff pastry	370 g	$3.83			
Final pie	1300 g	$16.91		1100 g	$14.30

Pie pastry

When we had our training wheels on we used to buy butter puff pastry, but we don't do that anymore (and it's not just because it would save us $4 per pie). Butter puff is now harder to find and getting more expensive by the day. This recipe makes three sheets. You only need two for the pie. Lizzie will often use the third to make swirls (see below) or other treats (such as making an apple turnover with stewed apple and cinnamon). Alternatively you could double this recipe and get two extra pies worth of pastry to put in your freezer for the next time the meat pie urge takes you.

Makes 3 sheets (standard supermarket sizing)

INGREDIENTS
2½ cups plain flour, plus extra for dusting
1 tablespoon dextrose (optional)
1 teaspoon salt
225 g unsalted butter, cut into 1 cm or smaller cubes (or, even better, grated)
1 cup very cold water (you may not need all of this)

METHOD
1. Mix the flour, dextrose (if using) and salt in a large bowl.
2. The most important thing with pastry is to keep everything cool. After cutting the butter, put it back in the fridge until just before you need it. Cold butter works best.
3. Sprinkle your butter cubes over your dry mix and begin to work them in with your pastry blender (or fingertips). Remember to be patient; you want the butter pieces the size of tiny peas throughout your dough. If you've grated the butter this step is easier.
4. Drizzle half the water into the flour/butter mix, gathering the dough together with a rubber or silicone spatula (or your fingers).
5. When the water is incorporated, add a little more at a time until the dough just comes together.

6. Once you have large clumps of pastry, use your hands to gently form your dough into a single piece.

7. Divide the dough into two pieces (I make one slightly larger than the other for the base of the pie). Place each on a separate piece of cling wrap and wrap the dough, using the sides of the cling wrap to press and shape the dough into a disc as you go. Place wrapped dough in the fridge for 1 hour (or even better 2, but we rarely have time).

8. When ready to roll out your pastry, flour your board and rolling pin. Make sure you have a template for the size you need your pastry to roll out to. And go gently; you want to keep those visible lumps of butter in the finished product.

9. There'll be a little bit of leftover pastry. You could use that to decorate the pie or you could make a great little extra treat. Roll out the leftovers, spread them with strawberry jam (or leftover cream cheese icing or even Vegemite and cheese), roll them up and then cut them into scrolls. Lay them on a baking tray, bake until golden, and you'll have great little scrolls that taste yummy fresh and freeze well.

COSTINGS

Ingredients	Weight/ Volume	Cost	Processed alternative	Weight	Cost
2½ cups plain flour	325 g	$0.24	Pampas Butter Puff Pastry (3 pack): Wheat flour, unsalted butter (25%) (milk), water, salt, food acids (300, 330)	550 g	$5.72
1 tablespoon dextrose (optional)	9.6 g	$0.03			
1 teaspoon salt	5.7 g	$0.01			
225 grams unsalted butter	225 g	$1.34			
1 cup very cold water	250 ml	$0.00			
Final pastry	550 g	$1.62		550 g	$5.72

Hot chips from scratch

This might seem like a lot of people to feed with a kilo of potatoes but this is not the meal, it's part of the meal. This is meant to replace the amount of potato you might provide by any other method (e.g. mashing or roasting). And once you've gone to all this trouble you want people to savour your boutique chippies rather than wolf them down like cow-fodder.

Serves 4 adults and 4 children

INGREDIENTS
washed potatoes (allow at least one large potato per person)
2 kg solidified cooking oil (we use Supafry) or 2 litres refined
    (extra light/mild) olive oil
salt, to taste
vinegar, to taste (optional)

METHOD
1. Peel the potatoes (you can leave the skins on if you want them American-style). Cut into chip shapes; this is immeasurably easier if you get a potato chipper from your local kitchenware store.
2. Parboil chips until soft when pricked with a fork (usually 5–10 minutes, depending on size) but not so soft that they break apart.
3. Dry (with paper towel) and cool (preferably in the fridge or freezer).
4. Put enough fat to cover the potatoes in deep-fryer and turn to 80 per cent of maximum heat (about 160°C).
5. After checking that the cooking fat has reached the set heat, deep-fry (using the chip basket if you have one) until a little colour starts to appear.
6. Retrieve the chips from the fat (this is where it's good to have a chip basket or some sort of sieve) and place them onto paper towel. Allow them to cool back to room temperature (should take about 15–20 minutes).
7. Deep-fry chips again at full heat (190–200°C) until golden brown.
8. Once again retrieve the chips from the fat and place them on clean paper towel, then add salt (and vinegar, if you like) to taste.

Pro-Tip: You can freeze the chips after the first frying. When I want chips I want them now! You can short-circuit this process by batching up a big load of chips after the first frying. Once they've cooled, place the chips in a plastic freezer bag in the portion sizes you're likely to need. Then, when you want to use them, pull them out and do the final fry (no need to thaw first). They'll stick together when you take them out of the freezer but don't worry, they will separate in the fryer.

COSTINGS

Ingredients	Weight/ Volume	Cost	Processed alternative	Weight	Cost
washed potatoes	1 kg	$3.98	McCain Healthy Choice Straight Cut Frozen Potato Chips: Potato (97%), canola oil, dextrose (maize)	1 kg	$4.50
2 kg solidified cooking oil (we use Supafry) or 2 litres refined (extra light/mild) olive oil (Note: you'll be using this at least four times so I've divided the cost by four)	2 kg	$3.14			
Final chips	1 kg	$7.12		1 kg	$4.50

Can't be bothered chips

Serves 4 adults and 4 children

INGREDIENTS

2 kg solidified cooking oil (we use Supafry) or 2 litres refined (extra light/mild) olive oil

1 kg McCain Healthy Choice Straight Cut Frozen Potato Chips (yes, there's some canola, but if this is all the exposure you get in a week, it's not going to do any real harm)

METHOD

1. Put appropriate amount of fat in deep-fryer and turn to maximum heat (190–200°C).
2. Deep-fry chips at full heat until golden-brown. Most fryers have a 2-litre capacity for oil so you'll only be able to fry about half a bag (500 g) at a time.
3. Retrieve the chips from the fat and place onto paper towel and season to taste.

Something to do with breadcrumbs

Due to overwhelming demand from his siblings, my eldest son, Anthony, developed this crumb recipe, which his little sister Finlayson whips up every now and then as part of her 'deep-fried dinner'.

Crumbing shortens the life of your cooking oil. You'll get fewer cycles out of it if you're crumbing each time because the crumbs dirty the oil much more than a batter or chips alone.

Deep-fried dinner crumbs

Because the chicken is being bashed flat this turns into quite a lot of servings (3 breasts would normally just feed a family of four). So if you're not cooking for eight, consider either halving the recipe or thinking about serving some nice crumbed chicken fillet sandwiches for school or work lunches for the rest of the week. The cooked fillets store well in the fridge and can be reheated in a frying pan.

Serves 4 adults and 4 kids (makes enough crumbs for three half chicken breasts or about 1 kg chicken)

INGREDIENTS*

2 teaspoons black peppercorns

1 tablespoon mixed herbs (dried or fresh)

1½ teaspoons salt

2¼ cups fresh breadcrumbs (see page 240)

4 eggs

¾ cup plain flour

*   To use the breadcrumbs as per the method below, you'll also need saturated fat for deep-frying and a food to be deep-fried.

METHOD

1. Place fat in fryer and turn to maximum heat (about 200°C).
2. Combine peppercorns, herbs and salt in a mortar and pestle, and grind finely.
3. In a bowl, combine the ground mixture with breadcrumbs by hand.
4. In a separate bowl, whisk eggs.
5. Sift flour into another bowl.
6. Line up your ingredients in this order: food to be deep-fried, bowl of flour, bowl of egg, bowl of crumb mixture, then deep-fryer.
7. Designate a dry hand (say, your left) and a wet hand (say, your right).
8. With your dry hand, roll the food in the flour, making sure it's well coated. Try to avoid having any bits which aren't covered in flour.
9. Continuing with your dry hand, place the food into the egg, then retrieve it using your wet hand. Hold the food over the egg bowl to drain off any excess.
10. Continuing with your wet hand, roll the food in the crumb mix and cover it well (once again, no gaps) before removing it.

11. Now, still with your wet hand, hold the food by one end and slowly lower it into the hot fat. Don't just throw it in, because this will cause the fat to spatter and the crumbs will fall off.

12. Fry until golden-brown. You'll know it's cooked when it begins to float (raw meat sinks to the bottom of the fryer but cooked meat floats). Once it's cooked pull it out of the fat with the fryer basket, a slotted spoon or tongs and drip-dry over the fat.

13. Drain the cooked food on a wire rack. The drips can be messy so it's a good idea to put some paper towel under the rack first.

COSTINGS

Ingredients	Weight/Volume	Cost	Processed alternative	Weight	Cost
2 teaspoons black peppercorns	11 g	$0.60	Tandaco Coating Mix for Southern Fried Chicken (8 packs of 75 g): Wheat flour, breadcrumbs (cereals and cereal flours [wheat, rye, soy, barley], water, yeast, iodised salt, vinegar, vegetable oil, emulsifiers [481, 471, 472e], preservative [282], vitamins [thiamine, folic acid]), starch (wheat and maize), salt, maltodextrin, spices (2%), flavour, sugar, baking powder, herbs (0.8%), vegetable gum (guar)	600 g	$16.00
1 tablespoon mixed herbs	9.6 g	$0.03			
1½ teaspoons salt	8 g	$0.01			
2¼ cups breadcrumbs	300 g	$0.40			
4 eggs	240 g	$1.68			
¾ cup plain flour	100 g	$0.08			
Final crumbs	600 g	$2.80		600 g	$16.00

Vegetables

The easy way to cook vegetables is to peel and cut them, then throw them into boiling water (or steam them) until they're soft enough to cut with a fork (or harder if you prefer). But if you want to do something a little fancier every now and then, here are a few recipes we use all the time.

Potato dauphinoise (potato bake)

This one is a strong favourite with the kids and beats mash every single time.

Serves 8 as side dish

INGREDIENTS

225 ml milk
1 cup cream
1 large clove (or 2 small cloves) garlic
2 sprigs of thyme
8 large washed potatoes
1 small sweet potato (optional)
salt and pepper, to taste
sprinkle of grated parmesan cheese

METHOD

1. Preheat oven to 200°C (most recipes suggest 180°C, but we usually cook it with our roast dinner at the temperature we use for roast beef – and it works) and generously grease an oven dish with butter.
2. Place milk, cream, garlic and thyme in a saucepan over medium heat to infuse the liquid with the flavours.
3. Cut the potatoes (skin on) and sweet potato into thin slices (scallops) – use a mandolin if you have one – it makes it dead easy.
4. Arrange your potato slices in the bottom of the dish, partly covering each row with the next so the base ends up looking like it's covered in fish scales.

5. Pour some of your milk sauce over the top (remove the garlic and thyme first) – not much, just enough to wet each of the slices.

6. Repeat this over and over until you run out of potatoes. Finish with a layer of sweet potato.

7. Pour the last of your milk mix over the top, season with salt and pepper, and sprinkle with parmesan cheese.

8. Cover your dish with foil and place in the oven for 45 minutes, then remove the foil and bake for another 30 minutes or until the top is crisp.

COSTINGS

Ingredients	Weight/ Volume	Cost	Processed alternative	Weight	Cost
225 ml milk	225 ml	$0.23	225 ml milk	225 ml	$0.23
1 cup cream	235 ml	$1.20	1 cup cream	235 ml	$1.20
1 large clove garlic (or 2 small)	10 g	$0.12	McCormick Produce Partners Scalloped Potato Recipe Base (2 packs of 40 g): Wheat flour, thickener (1422), salt, maltodextrin, onion, beverage whitener [(vegetable fat, glucose syrup solids, milk protein, emulsifiers (472e), mineral salts (340, 451), riboflavin, anti-caking agent (554)], sugar, yeast extract, soy bean oil, parsley, garlic, spice, vegetable gum (415), colour (150c)	80 g	$3.48
2 sprigs of thyme	1 g	$0.10			
8 large washed potatoes	1.3 kg	$5.15			
1 small sweet potato (optional)	300 g	$1.20			
salt and pepper, to taste	2 g	$0.01			
sprinkle of grated parmesan cheese	25 g	$0.68			
			8 large washed potatoes	1.3 kg	$5.15
			1 small sweet potato (optional)	300 g	$1.20
Final potato bake	1.9 kg	$8.69		1.9 kg	$11.26

Cauliflower au gratin

There aren't a lot of cauliflower fans at our place, but this one turns it from something to be avoided into the first thing eaten on the plate.

Serves 8 as side dish

INGREDIENTS
1 small head cauliflower, cut into florets
1 tablespoon butter, plus extra for greasing
1 tablespoon flour
¾ cup milk
salt and pepper, to taste
40 g tasty cheese, grated

METHOD
1. Preheat oven to 200°C and grease an ovenproof dish with butter.
2. Break cauliflower into florets and steam until tender (about 10 minutes).
3. Melt butter in a pan over moderate heat.
4. Add flour while stirring.
5. Add ¼ cup milk, whisking until smooth, then add another ¼ cup, whisking until smooth.
6. Keep whisking and allow the mixture to come to the boil. Keep whisking until it has the consistency of a thick gravy.
7. Remove from the heat, then add salt, pepper and half the cheese plus the last of the milk.
8. You should now have a pourable white sauce (which can be used for just about anything from fish to broccoli and everything in between).
9. Place your cauliflower florets neatly in one layer in the greased dish and pour all the sauce over the top.
10. Sprinkle with the remaining cheese.
11. Bake until the cheese browns (10–15 minutes).

COSTINGS

Ingredients	Weight/ Volume	Cost	Processed alternative	Weight	Cost
1 small head cauliflower	1300 g	$3.98	Birds Eye SteamFresh Cauliflower with Cheese Sauce (3 packs of 400 g): Cauliflower (55%), cream (14%), water, cheese (12%) (Emmental cheese [milk, salt, lactic culture, rennet], fresh cheese), skim milk powder, seasoning (contains egg), starch, garlic Note: There's nothing wrong with these ingredients; if you'd prefer to just buy this instead. It will take 3.5 minutes in the microwave.	1.2 kg	$13.20
1 tablespoon butter, plus extra for greasing	14 g	$0.08			
1 tablespoon flour	7.8 g	$0.01			
¾ cup milk	187 ml	$0.19			
salt and pepper, to taste	2 g	$0.01			
40 g tasty cheese	40 g	$0.70			
Final dish	1.4 kg	$4.97		1.2 kg	$13.20

Ratatouille

This is a great one to make up as a batch and have in the fridge. It's also useful because you get to use cheaper vegetables when out-of-season favourites are too pricey. Because you're baking them, the vegetables don't need to be perfect, which allows you to adjust quantities and types of vegetable based on cost (if you wish). If you can't be bothered whipping up vegetables as part of a meal, just scoop out some ratatouille and heat it for instant vegetables. It also goes well on a nice bit of buttered sourdough toast with some parmesan cheese or (our favourite) grilled haloumi.

Serves 8 as side dish

INGREDIENTS
6 tomatoes (Roma are best for this)
1 eggplant
2 zucchini
2 red onions
1 red capsicum
1 large clove (or 2 small cloves) garlic, finely chopped
sprigs of thyme or rosemary or whatever you can get your hands on

METHOD
1. Preheat oven to 200°C and grease a large baking tray with olive oil.
2. Cut tomatoes into 8 wedges each.
3. Cut other vegetables so they're approximately the size of the tomato wedges.
4. Add all the ingredients to the tray randomly, leaving the tomatoes till last.
5. Bake for 45 minutes or until vegies are tender.
6. Store in a sealed container in fridge, where it will last up to 2 weeks.

COSTINGS

Ingredients	Weight/ Volume	Cost	Processed alternative	Weight	Cost
6 tomatoes	600 g	$4.80	There isn't one		
1 eggplant	500 g	$3.99			
2 zucchini	420 g	$2.52			
2 red onions	400 g	$1.60			
1 red capsicum	320 g	$2.20			
1 large clove (or 2 small cloves) garlic	10 g	$0.12			
sprigs of thyme or rosemary		$0.50			
Final ratatouille	1.5 kg	$15.73			

* Remember, this is the absolute maximum this should cost. If you choose carefully, it will be considerably cheaper.

Condiments

Anthony's mayonnaise

We have daughters who love their chicken, lettuce and mayo rolls for school lunches. When we discovered there's no such thing (at least not in our local supermarkets) as mayo made without seed oil, we were in big trouble. Luckily, it turns out mayo isn't hard to make. Our eldest son, Anthony, doesn't do much in the house (he's at uni, so terribly 'busy'). But one thing he absolutely must do every week (or face a lynch party formed by his younger sisters) is make the mayo. He's gotten so good, he doesn't measure anything and it takes him slightly less time than waiting for his computer to turn on.

Makes 660 g (a large mayo bottle's worth)

INGREDIENTS

2 whole eggs (we prefer whole eggs – it's a great mayo and it avoids waste)

1 tablespoon Dijon mustard (we use Maille as it has no added sugar)

2 tablespoons lemon juice

2 cups refined (light/mild) olive oil

salt and pepper, to taste

METHOD

1. In a food processor (or with a whisk), pulse eggs, mustard and lemon juice.
2. Slowly (while processing) add olive oil until mixture thickens.
3. Taste and season if required.
4. Transfer to a sealed container and refrigerate.

This is a basic mayo recipe, but you can do endless variations by adding in 'flavourings'. If you want aioli, just add a couple of crushed garlic cloves, a dessertspoonful of lemon juice and a pinch of salt to a cup of mayo. To turn it into tartare sauce, to one cup of mayo add 1 tablespoon of finely chopped small onion, 2 chopped dill pickles (or some chopped gherkin), a splash of lemon juice, 1 tablespoon chopped fresh parsley, 1 teaspoon chives, and salt and pepper to taste.

COSTINGS

Ingredients	Weight/ Volume	Cost	Processed alternative	Weight	Cost
2 whole eggs	120 g	$0.84	Praise Whole Egg Creamy Mayonnaise: Sunflower oil (antioxidant [320]), whole egg (5%), egg yolk, water, white vinegar, cane sugar, lemon juice, Dijon-style mustard (food acid [acetic], colour [caramel III]), salt, garlic	670 g	$7.57
1 tablespoon Dijon mustard	18 g	$0.37			
2 tablespoons lemon juice	30 ml	$0.10			
2 cups refined olive oil	500 ml	$3.50			
salt and pepper, to taste	2 g	$0.01			
Final mayonnaise	660 g	$4.82		670 g	$7.57

Pizza sauce

Makes enough for 10 pizza bases (see recipe on page 236)

INGREDIENTS
1 large clove (or 2 small cloves) garlic
3 or 4 basil leaves (or sprigs of thyme or whatever herb you've got)
700 ml (1 bottle) tomato passata
salt and pepper, to taste

METHOD
1. Cut garlic into four pieces and rip up the basil leaves.
2. Pour passata into a saucepan and add garlic and basil leaves.
3. Warm passata gently until it just starts to boil, then remove from heat.
4. Remove the garlic and leaves and spread sauce over pizza bases with the back of a large spoon.

COSTINGS

Ingredients	Weight/ Volume	Cost	Processed alternative	Weight	Cost
1 large clove (or 2 small cloves) garlic	10 g	$0.12	Leggo's Squeeze Pizza Sauce (2 bottles of 400 g): Concentrated tomato (93%), onion (2.5%), garlic (2.5%), salt, garlic, herbs and spices, antioxidant (ascorbic acid), preservatives (202, 234 [contains barley])	800 g	$7.60
3 or 4 basil leaves	10 g	$0.10			
700 ml (1 bottle) tomato passata	700 ml	$3.52			
salt and pepper, to taste	2 g	$0.01			
Final sauce	800 g	$3.75		800 g	$7.60

Simple tomato sauce

Makes 500 g

INGREDIENTS

¼ cup extra virgin olive oil

2 large brown onions

1 large clove (or 2 small cloves) garlic

1 kg tomatoes

½ red capsicum

salt and pepper, to taste

METHOD

1. Heat oil in a saucepan over medium heat.
2. Dice onions and add to pan. Fry until they begin to colour.
3. Crush garlic and add to pan.
4. Roughly chop tomatoes and add to pan (the smaller the pieces, the faster they'll cook).
5. Dice capsicum and add to pan.
6. Cover and cook until well stewed (about 20 minutes).
7. Remove lid, reduce heat to a simmer and cook the sauce down, stirring occasionally (to stop it catching on bottom of pan).
8. After about 1 hour you should have a deep-red thick sauce.
9. Season to taste, remove from heat and, when cool, blend with a stick mixer or blender to remove any chunks (if desired).
10. Decant into suitable container and store in the fridge (also freezes well).

COSTINGS

Ingredients	Weight/ Volume	Cost	Processed alternative	Weight	Cost
¼ cup extra virgin olive oil	62.5 ml	$0.44	Dolmio Extra Garlic Pasta Sauce: Tomatoes 85% (from purée), garlic 8% (from chopped and roasted), sugar, onion, salt, basil, food acid (citric), yeast extract, pepper, paprika, oregano, fennel, garlic extract 0.5%	500 g	$3.62
2 large brown onions	360 g	$1.08			
1 large clove (or 2 small cloves) garlic	10 g	$0.12			
1 kg tomatoes	1 kg	$6.98*			
½ red capsicum	160 g	$1.10			
salt and pepper, to taste	2 g	$0.01			
Final sauce	500 g	$9.73		500 g	$3.62

*   This is full retail price for perfect eating tomatoes. You're going to chop them up and boil them, so you needn't go to the top shelf. Our local fruit shop does bags of overripe tomatoes for $2 a kilo. They often also do the same with capsicums. We use them and they're perfect for the job. Buy carefully with this primary ingredient, make in bulk and freeze, and the cost of this sauce and the dishes you make with it will plummet.

Baked beans

Now you have a sauce, what better thing to do with it than turn it into baked beans! They make a terrific, fast, nutritious hot breakfast, especially when you whack them on a bit of your freshly baked sourdough with butter.

Serves 4

INGREDIENTS
1 cup tomato sauce (see recipe above)
1 × 400 g can cannellini beans (or navy beans if you can find them)

METHOD
1. Mix beans and sauce in a saucepan and heat through over medium heat.
2. Serve.

COSTINGS

Ingredients	Weight/Volume	Cost	Processed alternative	Weight	Cost
1 cup tomato sauce	250 ml	$3.93	Heinz Baked Beans in Tomato Sauce (4 cans of 130 g): Navy beans (55%), tomato sauce (45%) (tomatoes [26%], water, sugar, maize thickener [1422], salt, food acid [acetic acid], flavours)	520 g	$4.28
1 × 400 g can cannellini beans	400 g	$1.10			
Final beans	520 g	$5.03		520 g	$4.28

Chunky multipurpose tomato sauce

This sauce uses the same basic recipe as the simple tomato sauce above, but adds some extra ingredients for flavour and texture, and you don't turn it into a smooth purée.

We make it about once a week. The beauty of this sauce is that it can accompany any vegetables in a main meal, is lovely with gnocchi and, if you throw in some pan-fried mince, you have a great bolognese sauce for a quick weekend meal. Even better, you can chuck some water, pasta, potato and carrot into the leftover bolognese sauce and you have minestrone soup. This thing is the Swiss army knife of quick meals, and it's very handy to have a batch ready to go in the fridge at all times. You can also adjust this recipe to match the seasonality (and therefore price) of the ingredients. Everything other than the tomatoes and onions is optional and can be altered according to what you have left over or what's on special.

Once again, I'm using comparison prices for full-cost perfect vegetables. You'd be nuts to pay these prices. You're going to stew this stuff, so what it looks like is irrelevant – head for the seconds bin and the prices will plummet.

This is a double recipe, meaning double what we'd normally make, but it's done this way to avoid leaving you with half an eggplant. The good news is this sauce freezes quite well, so consider dividing it in half (or lots of little bits) and freezing some.

Makes 2 kg

INGREDIENTS

1 eggplant
salt and pepper, to taste
½ cup extra virgin olive oil
2 large brown onions
2 large cloves (or 4 small cloves) garlic
2 kg tomatoes
1 red capsicum
2 celery stalks, leaves and all
2 tablespoons dried sumac spice (optional)
1 teaspoon chilli flakes (optional), to taste
200 g spinach leaves (frozen is just as good)
sprigs of oregano, thyme, parsley or chives, or whatever you have
    available (consider growing these yourself)

METHOD

1. Cut eggplant into top-to-bottom slices about 5 mm thick. Lay the
   slices on kitchen towel and cover generously with cooking salt.
   After 10 minutes wipe the salt and water off the slices then fry the
   pieces in a hot pan with a generous amount of the oil. Remove
   them from the heat once they colour.
2. Turn the pan down to medium heat and add some more oil.
3. Dice onions and add to pan. Fry until they begin to colour.
4. Crush garlic and add to pan.
5. Roughly chop tomatoes and add to pan.
6. Dice capsicum and add to pan.
7. Slice the celery crossways and add to pan with sumac and chilli
   flakes (if using).
8. Cover and cook until well stewed (about 20 minutes).
9. Roughly chop eggplant and add it with spinach, herbs and
   pepper, and a little salt to taste.
10. Reduce temperature so that the stew is just simmering and cook it
    down, stirring occasionally (to stop it catching on bottom of pan).
11. After about 1 hour you should have a deep-red thick sauce with
    some still recognisable chunks in the sauce.
12. Remove from heat and, when cool, store in the fridge in a lidded pot,
    ready to add to whatever 'fast food' you need to make that week.

COSTINGS

Ingredients	Weight/Volume	Cost	Processed alternative	Weight	Cost
1 eggplant	500 g	$3.99	Leggo's Bolognese Chunky Pasta Sauce (3 bottles of 750 g): Tomatoes (81%) (reconstituted, paste, diced), vegetables (onion, carrot, garlic, red capsicum), canola oil, sugar, thickener (1442), salt, yeast extract, parmesan cheese (contains milk), herbs, spices, food acid (citric), natural colour (paprika oleoresins)	2.25 kg	$13.53
½ cup extra virgin olive oil	125 ml	$0.86			
2 large brown onions	360 g	$1.08			
2 large cloves (or 4 small cloves) garlic	20 g	$0.24			
2 kg tomatoes	2000 g	$13.96			
1 red capsicum	320 g	$2.20			
2 celery stalks, leaves and all	200 g	$0.34			
2 tablespoons dried sumac spice (optional)	15 g	$1.12			
1 teaspoon chilli flakes (optional)	1.5 g	$0.16			
200 g spinach leaves	200 g	$3.40			
sprigs of oregano, thyme, parsley or chives	15 g	$1.20			
salt and pepper, to taste	2 g	$0.01			
Final sauce	2 kg	$28.56		2.25 kg	$13.53

Sweet treats

Ingredients

In these recipes you'll be using a couple of ingredients repeatedly – buttermilk and vanilla. Both are expensive if you buy them commercially and may contain undesirable ingredients (such as skim milk or sugar). The other big problem is waste. If you buy buttermilk you need to get it in multiples of 600 ml. That's great if that's exactly what you need but means you'll be tossing out an expensive ingredient if it isn't (you won't be putting this stuff on your porridge). If you make it yourself you make exactly what you need, no more, no less. This section sets out the simple recipes we use all the time.

Buttermilk

Lizzie often uses buttermilk instead of milk when she wants the end result to be fluffier and lighter. If light and fluffy is what you're after, just substitute buttermilk one for one wherever a recipe calls for milk. This is the recipe we use if we have yoghurt on hand. But if you don't, you could use sour cream instead and it will still work.

Makes 1 cup

INGREDIENTS
¾ cup Greek or plain yoghurt
¼ cup milk

METHOD
1. Mix yoghurt and milk together in a bowl with a fork or whisk until you have a smooth milky liquid.

COSTINGS

Ingredients	Weight/Volume	Cost	Processed alternative	Weight	Cost
¾ cup Greek or plain yoghurt	194 g	$1.37	Dairy Farmers Buttermilk: Skim milk, milk, concentrated skim milk, culture (but remember you will need to buy 600 ml minimum)	250 ml	$1.12
¼ cup milk	62 ml	$0.06			
Final buttermilk	250 ml	$1.43		250 ml	$1.12

Vanilla essence

Vanilla fools sugar-hungry tastebuds. It doesn't make things any sweeter, but as soon as you add vanilla it *seems* sweeter. We make our own. You don't have to but it's extraordinarily easy to do and if you buy the beans and vodka in bulk you'll have a constant, relatively inexpensive supply. The prices below (and in all the recipes) are based on full retail pricing. You can probably do a lot better than that for these ingredients. We bought our beans in bulk on the internet, waited for a vodka sale, found some nice bottles, made as much as we needed and gave the rest away as gifts. This recipe has a bit of a lead time (it will be three months before you have a usable batch) but it's worth it once you get going (because you can have a constant supply).

Makes 200 ml

INGREDIENTS
2 large vanilla beans
200 ml vodka

METHOD
1. Find a small (200 ml) bottle you can seal (old Moccona coffee jars are good for this).
2. Cut beans in half lengthways, then carefully use the point of the knife to scrape out the seeds. Place the seeds in the bottle along with the dissected beans.
3. Fill bottle with vodka.
4. Leave in a cool dark place for 3 months.
5. When the bottle is about half-empty you can just add more vodka. If the flavour gets too weak, throw in another bean with the extra vodka.

Ingredients	Weight/ Volume	Cost	Processed alternative	Weight	Cost
2 large dried vanilla beans	8 g	$2.30	Queen Natural Organic Vanilla Extract (2 bottles of 100 ml): Extract of organic vanilla beans (water, organic alcohol [35%], organic sugar)	200 ml	$13.76
200 ml vodka	200 ml	$8.57			
Final essence	200 ml	$10.87		200 ml	$13.76

Vanilla yoghurt

Let's start simple. A lot of people struggle with the tartness of Greek (or plain) yoghurt when they first stop eating processed food. But a great way to take the edge off is to add some vanilla or even stir through a little dextrose. Kids love that as a treat, and it's nothing but good for them. And it tastes magnificent poured over fruit salad with some toasted coconut and almond slivers.

TV chocolate slice

A few years ago a TV crew came to our house and asked me to 'make something' for the cameras. Since the entire extent of my baking capabilities is, well, toast, I was in a bit of a pickle. Lizzie thought quickly and came up with this chocolate slice. The TV crew said not to worry, no one could taste it through the telly, so I should just go for it. After the shoot, I was ready to bin it, but Lizzie said we should whack it in the oven and see what it was like. We did and after trying a new icing (that Lizzie had been experimenting with) on it, it turned out magnificently. In fact, it's so popular with our kids that Lizzie cooks this one at least once a week. It's a real lunch-box favourite. So here it is – TV Chocolate Slice – so easy even I can make it!

This recipe also works well with gluten-free flour

Makes 1 medium tray (24 large pieces)

INGREDIENTS

Slice

1¾ cups plain flour

¼ cup cocoa

1 cup dextrose

200 g butter, melted and cooled

Icing

1 cup dextrose

1 tablespoon cocoa

20 g butter

1 tablespoon cream

METHOD

To make the slice:

1. Preheat oven to 180°C and line an 18.5 × 28.5 cm slice tin with baking paper.
2. Mix all dry ingredients together.
3. Add butter and stir, then knead to combine.
4. Press into lined tin.
5. Bake for 15 minutes.
6. Cut while still warm.
7. Ice when cool.

To make the icing:

1. Place all ingredients except cream in a bowl over a saucepan of water simmering on the stove (or you can place directly in a saucepan over a low heat, but you don't want the dextrose to boil and therefore become a toffee, or the icing won't set).
2. Allow dextrose to dissolve and combine with the other ingredients – heat but don't boil.
3. Add cream then remove from the heat to cool slightly and thicken.
4. Using a knife, spread evenly over the slice.
5. Allow to set at room temperature – then store in the fridge or freezer (it tastes great cold but lasts well in the lunch-box, too).

COSTINGS

Ingredients	Weight/ Volume	Cost	Processed alternative	Weight	Cost
Slice					
1¾ cups plain flour	230 g	$0.17	Coles Double Chocolate Chip Cookies (3 packs of 12 [264 g]): Wheat flour, sugar, vegetable margarine (vegetable fats and oils [palm, canola, coconut], water, salt, emulsifiers [322 (soy), 471], antioxidant [306 (soy)], colours [100, 160b]), dark compound choc chips (9%) (sugar, vegetable fat [palm], cocoa powder, emulsifiers [322 (soy), 492], milk solids), cocoa powder (5.8%), glucose (contains preservative [220]), milk solids, raising agent (450, 500, 541), vegetable oil (canola), salt, natural flavour, egg powder	792 g	$10.05
¼ cup cocoa	31 g	$0.79			
1 cup dextrose	162 g	$0.58			
200 g butter	200 g	$1.19			
Icing					
1 cup dextrose	162 g	$0.58			
1 tablespoon cocoa	7.4 g	$0.10			
20 g butter	20 g	$0.12			
1 tablespoon cream	15 g	$0.08			
Final slice	800 g	$2.90		792 g	$10.05

Rice malt syrup snaps

Lizzie and I saw Matthew Evans (*The Gourmet Farmer*) whip up a batch of these simple biscuits on the telly one evening. It inspired me to ask Lizzie to give it a go with rice malt syrup. She did and they've become a regular feature in the bickie tin around here. They're quick and easy to make, and the kids love them in the lunch-box. They stay especially crispy if you store them in the freezer.

This recipe also works well with gluten-free flour

Makes 36 biscuits

INGREDIENTS
100 g butter
½ cup rice malt syrup
1 cup plain flour
¼ teaspoon bicarbonate of soda
¼ teaspoon ground ginger (or mixed spice) or ½ teaspoon cinnamon

METHOD
1. Preheat oven to 180°C and line two baking trays with paper.
2. Melt butter, adding rice malt syrup and stirring until combined (you don't want it to be too hot – ensure it's no more than lukewarm before you add flour).
3. Add flour, bicarbonate of soda and spice. Stir well until smooth (the consistency of a thick caramel sauce).
4. Place dessertspoonfuls of mix on the baking trays with enough space between for biscuits to spread without touching (although Lizzie easily snaps apart biscuits that have strayed).
5. Use your (wet – cos they don't stick) fingers or the back of a spoon to flatten mix (these biscuits are particularly lovely when thin and really crispy).
6. Bake for about 10 minutes (depending on thickness) until coloured but not dark (biscuits will harden as they cool).
7. Cool on tray until biscuits harden, then transfer to rack to cool completely.
8. Store in an airtight container. (We store ours in the freezer and they're even better the second day.)

COSTINGS

Ingredients	Weight/Volume	Cost	Processed alternative	Weight	Cost
100 g butter	100 g	$0.59	Arnott's Ginger Nut Biscuits (2 packs of 250 g): Wheat flour, sugar, golden syrup, vegetable oil (contains soy), baking powder, ginger, salt, flavour (natural)	500 g	$5.10
½ cup rice malt syrup	182 g	$1.44			
1 cup plain flour	132 g	$0.10			
¼ teaspoon bicarbonate of soda	1.1 g	$0.01			
¼ teaspoon ground ginger (or mixed spice) or ½ teaspoon cinnamon	1.1 g	$0.11			
Final biscuits	400 g	$2.26		500 g	$5.10

Pikelets and jam

Lizzie occasionally likes to whip up some afternoon tea for the hungry hordes descending from school, especially when they're bringing friends. This is a good recipe for a mixed audience of sugar eaters and non-sugar eaters, as sugar-free pikelets taste almost identical to the full-sugar variety. This is one of the kids' favourites. Even if Lizzie hasn't bothered with the jam, they still love them hot with lashings of butter.

Makes 16 large pikelets

INGREDIENTS
Pikelets
1 whole egg
3 tablespoons dextrose
¾ cup milk or buttermilk
1 cup self-raising flour
pinch of salt
1 tablespoon butter, melted, plus extra to grease the pan
Strawberry jam
1 punnet (250 g) strawberries (or frozen raspberries or blueberries)
2 tablespoons dextrose, or rice malt syrup, to taste (both optional –
    we no longer bother)

METHOD
To make the pikelets:
1. Whisk egg, dextrose and half the milk in a bowl until smooth.
2. Sift flour and salt into mix and combine.
3. Add rest of milk (aiming for a batter the consistency of thick cream).
4. Add melted butter.
5. Preheat and lightly grease a frying pan.
6. Working in batches, drop spoonfuls (the bigger the spoon you use, the bigger the pikelets you'll get) of batter into pan and cook until bubbles form on surface, then flip to cook other side.
7. Remove and wrap in a tea towel or napkin (to keep warm while you cook the next batch) before serving.

To make the jam:

1. Wash, hull and halve (or quarter depending on size) the strawberries.
2. Place in a lidded saucepan over a moderate heat for 5 minutes (approximately – don't leave unattended; the lid allows the fluid from the strawberries basically to boil them, so they can boil over).
3. Remove lid and lower temperature while stirring through dextrose, if using.
4. Cook down until enough fluid evaporates and you're left with a jam-like texture (with fruit chunks). The jam will thicken slightly as it cools.
5. Cool and serve.

COSTINGS

Ingredients	Weight/Volume	Cost	Processed alternative	Weight	Cost
Pikelets					
1 whole egg	60 g	$0.42	Golden Pikelets (2 packs of 8 pikelets): Water, wheat flour, sugar, canola oil, milk solids, acidity regulator (575), wheat starch, egg powder, raising agent (500), salt, preservatives (234, 202), emulsifier (471), flavour, colour (161b), vitamins (thiamine, folate)	400 g	$7.80
3 tablespoons dextrose	28.7 g	$0.09			
¾ cup milk or buttermilk	187 ml	$0.19			
1 cup self-raising flour	132 g	$0.10			
pinch of salt	0 g	$0.00			
1 tablespoon butter	14 g	$0.08			
Strawberry jam					
1 punnet strawberries or frozen raspberries or blueberries)	250 g	$1.98	IXL Strawberry Conserve: Sugar, strawberries (40%), gelling agent (fruit pectin), food acids (330, 331)	250 g	$2.81
2 tablespoons dextrose (optional)	19.2 g	$0.06			
Final dish	75 g	$2.89			$10.61

Strawberry clafoutis

Our local fruiterer often has a special on strawberries. We've found that if we buy them, process them (wash and trim them) and then freeze them we have a ready supply for whenever we need to knock up a quick dessert like this one (or make jam).

This recipe is one that most of the family loves. Clafoutis (traditionally made with cherries) cooks fruit in a pancake-like batter. Before you say ewww because of my clumsy description, know that it tastes great, especially served warm with thickened cream (whipped or just poured over it) on a cold winter's night (or morning for breakfast, for that matter). The fruit doesn't have to be pristine, as it's being baked, so it's a great way to enjoy those strawberries.

We've also cooked this dish using frozen raspberries. It was good but it made us wish we'd used strawberries. See what you think.

Serves 8

INGREDIENTS

2 eggs
80 g plain flour
80 g butter, melted and cooled
60 g dextrose (just over ⅓ cup)
150 ml milk
1 teaspoon vanilla essence
1 punnet (250 g) strawberries (or you could use frozen raspberries or blueberries) – if you have more strawberries at hand, 300 g is a better amount

METHOD

1. Preheat oven to 200°C and grease a 20 cm round baking dish.
2. Lightly beat eggs.
3. Add flour.

4. Whisk in butter.
5. Gradually mix in dextrose and milk.
6. Add vanilla.
7. Spread strawberries evenly over bottom of prepared dish.
8. Pour over batter and place in oven.
9. Bake for 10 minutes before reducing temperature to 180°C and baking for a further 25 minutes.
10. Serve warm with cream.

COSTINGS

Ingredients	Weight/Volume	Cost	Processed alternative	Weight	Cost
2 eggs	120 g	$0.84	Sara Lee Apple and Berry Pie with Crumble (yes, I know it's not the same thing, but it's as close as I could get): Apple (28%), wheat flour (thiamine), sugar, margarine [animal and vegetable fats and oils, water, salt, emulsifiers (471, soy lecithin, 472c), milk solids, natural flavour, antioxidant (306), citric acid, natural colour (carotene)], water, berries (5%) (blackberries, blueberries), thickener (1412), dextrose, whey powder, salt, vegetable gum (407), mineral salt (508), raising agents (450, sodium bicarbonate), citric acid. Crumble: 26%	600 g	$6.60
80 g plain flour	80 g	$0.06			
80 g butter	80 g	$0.48			
60 g dextrose	60 g	$0.22			
150 ml milk	150 ml	$0.15			
1 teaspoon vanilla essence	4.9 ml	$0.27			
1 punnet strawberries	250 g	$1.98			
Final clafoutis	600 g	$4.00		600 g	$6.60

Red velvet cupcakes

Real-food eaters need to live in the real world. Often that means having to turn up with something for an end-of-year school do or a cake stall. These little beauties fit the bill perfectly. They're simple to make, safe for you and your kids to eat, and sweet enough to be a hit with any fake-food eater.

You could easily leave out the colouring if using it concerns you (it will taste exactly the same), although the colour of the cakes does add somewhat to their allure.

Lizzie says this recipe is the one that taught her the value of buttermilk. It doesn't require that you own a benchtop mixer, so it's an equipment-lite recipe. And you can (and we have many times) easily turn it into a birthday or other celebration cake by using self-raising flour instead of plain flour, making two cakes (from this mix using 2 × 20 cm round tins), adjusting the cooking times and icing them in layers.

The cream cheese icing is reasonably stable – that is, it's not as affected by heat as a butter-based icing. Any leftover icing stores well in the fridge and can be frozen. Lizzie often adds cocoa to this and spreads it on leftover pastry to make scrolls (see page 234) or spreads it on the last pizza base with a sprinkle of coconut and slivered almonds to make what our kids have christened 'Pudza' (pudding pizza).

This recipe also works well with gluten-free flour

Makes 16–18 large cupcakes

Note though that we normally make 48 mini-cakes – which are terrific single serve treats with dextrose dusting rather than the icing. If we are cooking for sugar eaters (say as a bring-a-plate) then we will use the icing (which is quite sweet) to make butterfly cakes.

INGREDIENTS

Cakes

2 cups plain flour

¼ cup cocoa

1 teaspoon bicarbonate of soda

2 cups dextrose

2–3 teaspoons red food colouring (optional)

1 cup buttermilk

200 g unsalted butter, melted and cooled

3 eggs, lightly whisked

1 tablespoon white vinegar

1 teaspoon vanilla essence

Icing

120 g butter, softened

250 g cream cheese, at room temperature

pinch of salt

2 cups dextrose, or to taste (adjust for likely audience – you may get away with fewer tastes as you go), plus extra for dusting

2 teaspoons vanilla essence (optional)

METHOD

To make the cupcakes:

1. Preheat oven to 170°C and line a large muffin tray with large patty papers.
2. Sift flour, cocoa and bicarbonate of soda into a bowl.
3. Stir through dextrose.
4. Whisk colouring (if using), buttermilk, butter, eggs, vinegar and vanilla together.
5. Make a well in the dry ingredients. Add liquid ingredients and stir until combined.
6. Spoon mixture into the lined tray.
7. Bake for 20–25 minutes.
8. Cool on a wire rack.
9. These cakes freeze well.

To make the icing:

1. Beat butter, cream cheese and salt until smooth.
2. Add dextrose to taste, a little at a time.

3. Add vanilla (if using) and beat until mixture is smooth.
4. Spread icing over cakes with a knife or, if you want to get fancy and make butterfly cakes, dig a circle out of the top and cut it in half, insert a generous teaspoon of the icing and add the cut-out pieces as wings.
5. Dust with dextrose.
6. Serve fresh. Leftovers store well in the fridge.

COSTINGS

Ingredients	Weight/Volume	Cost	Processed alternative	Weight	Cost
Cakes					
2 cups plain flour	264 g	$0.20	Coles Red Velvet Swirl Cupcakes (4 x 4 pack): Red velvet sponge (75%): sugar, wheat flour, vegetable oil (canola), thickener (1422), egg powder, wheat starch, cocoa, raising agents (500, 541, 341, 450), salt, vegetable emulsifier (481), preservative (202), natural colour (120), water. Cream-cheese frosting (25%): icing sugar (sugar, maize starch), glucose, vegetable shortening (vegetable oil [palm, canola, coconut], vegetable emulsifier [471 (soy)], antioxidant [306 (soy)]), cream cheese (milk), cream cheese powder (milk), natural colour (150a), preservative (202), salt. Not suitable for vegetarians	960 g	$18.00
¼ cup cocoa	31 g	$0.79			
1 teaspoon bicarbonate of soda	4.6 g	$0.02			
2 cups dextrose	324 g	$1.16			
2–3 teaspoons red food colouring (optional)	14.8 ml	$0.36			
1 cup buttermilk	250 ml	$1.12			
200 g unsalted butter	200 g	$1.19			
3 eggs	180 g	$1.26			
1 tablespoon white vinegar	14.8 ml	$0.01			
1 teaspoon vanilla essence	4.9 ml	$0.27			

Ingredients	Weight/ Volume	Cost	Processed alternative	Weight	Cost
Icing					
120 g butter	120 g	$0.72			
250 g cream cheese	250 g	$4.34			
pinch of salt	0 g	$0.00			
2 cups dextrose	324 g	$1.16			
2 teaspoons vanilla essence (optional)	9.8 ml	$0.56			
Final cakes	1280 g	$13.16		1280 g	$18.00

Super custard

We call this recipe Super Custard because this one simple recipe can be used to make four different puddings: pouring custard, ice-cream, crème brûlée and baked custard. This isn't the normal way of making custard, but by massively simplifying the recipe (and particularly the method), Lizzie has created a quick, all-purpose dessert-making tool. There's nowhere near the fuss and chefs will be cringing as they read this recipe, but it works and it works well.

Master this puppy and you can be a dessert queen or king with just one recipe.

Pouring custard

This the base set of ingredients and recipe.

Serves 10

INGREDIENTS
600 ml cream
3 eggs
½ cup dextrose
300 ml milk
1 teaspoon vanilla essence

METHOD
1. Whisk all ingredients together in a bowl.
2. Pour into a saucepan over moderate heat, whisking continuously.
3. Allow to steam but not boil (while whisking).
4. Whisk until thickened (should be about 10 minutes).
5. Take off the heat and allow to cool. It will thicken as it cools.
6. Store in fridge until ready for use.

COSTINGS

Ingredients	Weight/ Volume	Cost	Processed alternative	Weight	Cost
600 ml cream	600 ml	$3.00	Dairy Farmers Vanilla Pouring Custard Milk, skim milk, sugar, thickener (1442 [corn]), concentrated skim milk, flavour, vegetable gums (407, 412, 415), natural colours (160a, 160b), mineral salt (452). Ultra-pasteurised	1 kg	$4.73
3 eggs	180 g	$1.26			
½ cup dextrose	80 g	$0.29			
300 ml milk	300 ml	$0.30			
1 teaspoon vanilla essence	4.9 ml	$0.27			
Final custard	1 kg	$5.12		1 kg	$4.73

Ice-cream

To make ice-cream instead, you'll need more dextrose and some glucose syrup. I've highlighted the changes in the ingredients list below.

Makes 1 litre

INGREDIENTS

600 ml cream

3 eggs

1 cup dextrose

300 ml milk

1 teaspoon vanilla essence

1 heaped tablespoon glucose syrup (optional – this stops it setting too hard)

If you want more than just vanilla ice-cream, use exactly the same recipe but:

For chocolate, add cocoa to taste (¼ to ⅓ cup).

For mocha, add cocoa and coffee (¼ to ⅓ cup cocoa plus 1 teaspoon instant coffee). If it's a bitter flavour, you might need some more dextrose – adjust to taste.

For strawberry, add some strawberry jam (see recipe on page 281).

For coffee, add brewed coffee to the mix.

METHOD

Make exactly as for pouring custard, but if you decide to use the glucose syrup, add it to the custard when it's warm in the saucepan, then:

1. If you don't have an ice-cream churner, place the mixture in a bowl in the freezer and pull it out every 1–2 hours and whisk. Keep doing this until it's completely frozen.

2. If you do have a churner, wait till the mixture is cooled, then churn it until you have a soft-serve ice-cream, then decant into an old ice-cream container and freeze.

3. Could it be any simpler?

COSTINGS

Ingredients	Weight/Volume	Cost	Processed alternative	Weight	Cost
600 ml cream	600 ml	$3.00	Peters Original Vanilla Ice Cream: Water, cream (15%), sugar, milk solids, glucose syrup (wheat), maltodextrin, vegetable origin emulsifiers (477, 471 [soy]), flavour, vegetable gum (412)	1 litre	$3.15
3 eggs	180 g	$1.26			
1 cup dextrose	162 g	$0.58			
300 ml milk	300 ml	$0.30			
1 teaspoon vanilla essence	4.9 ml	$0.27			
1 heaped tablespoon glucose syrup (optional)	21 g	$0.20			
Final ice-cream	1 litre	$5.61		1 litre	$3.15

Crème brûlée

To make crème brûlée instead, all you need do is revert to the original custard recipe. When they're done, make a hard-sugar top for a professional finish. To do this, cover the top of each with some dextrose and cook them under the grill or use a kitchen blowtorch to caramelise the dextrose.

Traditional recipes for crème brûlée will demand you use egg yolks rather than whole eggs, but this gets an almost identical result without all the waste.

METHOD
1. Preheat oven to 180°C.
2. Whisk all ingredients together thoroughly in a bowl or jug.
3. Pour the mixture into eight greased (with butter) small (150 ml) ramekins.
4. Cover ramekins with tin foil (a small sheet for each one, pressed down around the top of the ramekin). This stops a crust forming.
5. Place ramekins in bain-marie (fill a large baking dish with water and place ramekins in it – water should be no higher than mix inside ramekins) and bake for 1 hour.
6. Chill, then do your sugar tops (see above) just before serving.

Baked custard

To make this a baked custard, use half as much cream (300 ml rather than 600 ml) and you will need some nutmeg (optional) but otherwise make it in identical fashion to the crème brûlée.

METHOD

1. Preheat oven to 180°C.
2. Whisk all ingredients together thoroughly in a bowl or jug.
3. Pour the mixture into six greased (with butter) small (150 ml) ramekins.
4. Grate nutmeg (or sprinkle ground nutmeg) lightly over the top of each.
5. Place ramekins in bain-marie (fill a large baking dish with water and place ramekins in it – water should be no higher than mix inside ramekins) and bake for 40 minutes.
6. Chill before serving (and perhaps serve with some seasonal fruit).

SHOPPING LIST

Wouldn't it be great to know what type of fish or peanut butter or beef or spread to buy without having to spend hours looking through the book? Well, here's the shortcut. In the list that follows I've gathered together all my recommendations in one place, so you can spend more time doing what you do when you're not shopping. If it's not on this list then you shouldn't be buying it but it's always worth checking back to the relevant section, because I often provide work-arounds.

Sweeteners

- Corn syrup
- Dextrose
- Glucose
- Glucose syrup
- Lactose
- Maltose
- Maltodextrin
- Maltodextrose
- Rice malt syrup

Meat (if you eat meat)

- Whole, sliced or minced beef and lamb (grain fed if possible but don't stress if it's not)
- Whole, sliced or minced bacon and other pork products (grain fed if possible otherwise trim the fat)
- Poultry (no restrictions)
- Sausages, rissoles, crumbed filets and other pre-made meat and poultry products are usually fine, but check the ingredients list. If it contains sugar or 'vegetable oil' then avoid it. Be especially careful of crumbed products, soy flour is usually an ingredient as is vegetable oil.

Seafood

- Bream, oysters, tuna, cod, scallop, flathead, lobster, prawns and calamari (squid)
- Salmon if you know it's wild caught or farmed by Tassal in Tasmania
- Tinned fish only if it's tinned in water for example:
  - Coles Tuna Chunks in Springwater
  - John West Tuna in Springwater
  - Sirena Tuna in Springwater
  - Woolworths Select Tuna Tuna Chunks in Springwater
- If you must eat caviar choose red over black

Eggs (no restrictions)

Flours

- Barley
- Light rye
- Potato
- Rice
- Wheat

Pasta

- All dried or fresh pasta, couscous, quinoa and polenta sold without sauce

Breads

- Homemade
- Bürgen Rye
- Coles Smart Buy White
- Tip Top The One
- Tip Top Sunblest White
- Tip Top Up White + 25% Multigrain
- Most sourdough for example:
  - Bill's Organic Sourdough Olive Cobb
  - Coles Light Rye Sourdough Rolls
  - Coles Stone Baked White Sourdough Baguette
  - Coles White Sourdough Vienna
- European Varieties at bakeries for example:
  - Ciabatta
  - French sticks and rolls
  - Pasta Dura
  - BUT ask first, most of the chain bakeries (for example Baker's Delight and Brumby's) now use canola oil even in these traditional recipes

Wraps

- Mountain Bread brand
- Mission White Corn Tortillas
- Old El Paso Wholegrain Tortillas or Old El Paso Taco Shells

Unsweetened breakfast cereals and mueslis

- Abundant Earth Organic Puffed Corn
- Abundant Earth Organic Puffed Kamut
- Abundant Earth Organic Puffed Millet
- Abundant Earth Organic Puffed Rice
- Be Natural Porridge Original
- Biogenic Health Foods Yeast-free and Wheat-free Muesli
- Carman's Traditional Australian Oats
- Coles Oats Quick
- Coles Oats Rolled
- Coles Organic Bourghal
- Coles Organic Instant Oats
- Coles Organic Rolled Oats Creamy Style
- Coles Organic Rolled Oats Instant
- Coles Smart Buy Quick Oats Original
- Coles Smart Buy Rolled Oats
- Coles Smart Buy Wheat Biscuits Original
- Coles Whole Wheat Biscuits
- Flip Shelton's Natural Muesli (the one with just nuts and seeds)
- Food for Health Life Food The Fibre Cleanse Muesli
- Food for Health Life Food The Liver Cleansing Muesli
- Freedom Foods Quick Oats
- Golden Vale Minute Oats
- Golden Vale Wheat Biscuits
- Heartland Harvest Dry Roasted Muesli
- Lowan Quick Oats
- Lowan Rice Flakes

- Lowan Rolled Oats
- Quaker Oat So Simple Original
- Real Good Food Organic Fruit Free Muesli
- Sanitarium Puffed Wheat
- Sanitarium Weet-Bix Kids
- the muesli
- the muesli Gluten Free
- Uncle Toby's OatBrits
- Uncle Toby's Oats Multigrain
- Uncle Toby's Oats Quick
- Uncle Toby's Oats Traditional
- Uncle Toby's Oats Weightwise Original
- Uncle Toby's Shredded Wheat
- Uncle Toby's Vita Brits
- Uncle Toby's Vita Brits Weeties
- Woolworths Home Brand Quick Oats
- Woolworths Home Brand Rolled Oats
- Woolworths Home Brand Wheat Biscuits
- Woolworths Macro Natural Untoasted Muesli No added Fruit
- Woolworths Select Quick Cooking Oats
- Woolworths Select Rolled Oats

Whole fruit and berries

- Any whole berries but preferably strawberry, raspberry and blackberry
- Any whole fruit but preferably kiwi, fresh fig, orange, peach and apricot

Whole legumes, nuts and seeds

- Whole legumes such as beans and lentils are fine (canned is also fine). This doesn't include baked beans (because of the sugary sauce that comes with them)
- Any whole nuts but preferably chestnut, coconut, macadamia, hazelnut, cashew, almond, peanut and pistachio
- Avoid seeds unless being used as a garnish or flavouring

Whole vegetables (no restrictions)

Frozen Potato Products

- Birds Eye Curly Fries
- Birds Eye Steakhouse Chips
- Coles Steakhouse Chips
- McCain Healthy Choice Straight Cut
- McCain Healthy Choice Chunky Cut
- McCain Hot Bandito Wedges
- McCain Original Fries Crunchy Seasoned
- McCain Original Wedges Crunchy Seasoned
- McCain SuperFries Chunky Cut
- McCain SuperFries Mum's Cut
- McCain SuperFries Straight Cut

Crisps and Snacks

- Blackstone chips (plain only)
- Coles Corn Chips
- Doritos Original Corn Chips (plain only)
- Parkers Pretzels

- Red Rock Deli Sea Salt potato chips
- Smiths Extra Crunchy chips (plain only)

Cracker Biscuits

- Cruskits rye or corn
- Salada Multigrain 97% Fat Free
- Salada Light Original
- San-J Tamari Brown Rice Crackers

Butter (no restrictions)

If it comes from grass-fed animals then so much the better but it is not necessary.

Spreads

- Avocado
- Coles Brand Peanut Butter
- Sanitarium No Added Sugar or Salt Peanut Butter
- Macadamia Nut Butter
- Unflavoured cream cheese (any brand)
- Vegemite

Condiments

- Homemade olive oil mayonnaise, salad dressings & pestos
- Homemade tomato sauces
- Byron Bay Chilli Company Red Cayenne Chilli with Lime
- Byron Bay Chilli Company Green Jalapeno Chilli with Coriander
- Ayam or Squid Brand Fish Sauce

- Empower Foods LC Tomato (contains sucralose)
- Empower Foods LC Satay (contains sucralose)
- Kikkoman Soy Sauces
- Old El Paso Burrito Seasoning (best of a bad lot for this kind of condiment)

Unflavoured cream & milk (no restrictions)

Any whole full-fat milk or cream is fine as long as flavouring (e.g. chocolate) has not been added. If it comes from grass-fed animals then so much the better but it is not necessary.

Cheese (no restrictions)

Yoghurt

- Black Swan Greek Style Naturally Sweet
- Black Swan Greek Style Vanilla Bean
- Brooklea Lite Natural
- Chobani Low-Fat Plain
- Chobani Non-Fat Plain
- Coles Natural Set
- Farmers Union European Style Natural
- Farmers Union Greek Style Natural
- Five:am Natural No Added Sugar
- Gippsland Dairy Organic Natural
- Just Organic Natural
- Jalna a2 Low Fat Natural
- Jalna BioDynamic Organic Whole Milk
- Jalna Fat Free Natural

- Jalna Greek Low Fat Natural
- Jalna Greek Natural 4
- Jalna Leben European Style
- Jalna Premium Creamy Natural
- Liddells Lactose Free Plain
- Lyttos Lite Greek Style Natural
- Macro Wholefoods Market Organic Greek Style
- Nestlé Soleil Diet Black Cherry
- Nestlé Soleil Diet Fruit Salad
- Nestlé Soleil Diet Mixed Berry
- Nestlé Soleil Diet Passionfruit
- Nestlé Soleil Diet Peach & Mango
- Nestlé Soleil Diet Strawberry
- Nestlé Soleil Diet Vanilla
- Pauls All Natural 99.8% Fat Free
- Tamar Valley Greek Style No Added Sugar Mango
- Tamar Valley Greek Style No Added Sugar Mixed Berry
- Tamar Valley Greek Style No Added Sugar Raspberry
- Tamar Valley Greek Style No Added Sugar Strawberry
- Yoplait Formé Field Berries
- Yoplait Formé French Vanilla
- Yoplait Formé Peach Mango
- Yoplait Formé Passionfruit
- Yoplait Formé Raspberry
- Yoplait Formé Sticky Date
- Yoplait Formé Strawberry
- Yoplait Formé Tropical
- Woolworths Select Greek Style

Milk alternatives

- Limited amounts (really just for adding to tea or coffee) of any of:
    - Coles Lite Soy Milk
    - Vitasoy Lite
    - Sanitarium Lite
    - Sanitarium's So Good 99.9 % Fat Free
    - So Natural Rice Milk

Tea and coffee

This means the tea and coffee you make at home with a teabag or coffee. It does not include iced tea or coffee or those syrup-filled monstrosities you find in coffee shops.

Unflavoured water
Spirits
Beer

Dry wine

- White
    - Albariño
    - Chardonnay
    - Gewürztraminer
    - Grüner Veltliner
    - Muscadet
    - Sauvignon Blanc
    - Pinot Blanc
    - Pinot Grigio/Pinot Gris
    - Riesling
    - Viognier
- Champagne
    - Brut
    - Extra Brut
    - Extra Sec

- Red
  - Cabernet Sauvignon
  - Carménère
  - Cabernet Franc
  - Cinsaut
  - Grenache
  - Malbec
  - Marsanne
  - Merlot
  - Mouvedre
  - Petit Verdot
  - Pinot Noir
  - Roussanne
  - Sangiovese
  - Syrah
  - Viognier
  - Zinfandel
- Avoid any wine or champagne that has these words on the label:
  - Doce
  - Dolce
  - Demi-sec
  - Dessert
  - Dulce
  - Doux
  - Late harvest
  - Off-dry
  - Sec
  - Sweet

Fats

- Animal fat (includes lard, tallow, fowl fat etc)
- Avocado oil
- Butter
- Coconut oil
- Chestnut oil
- Ghee
- Macadamia nut oil
- Olive oil
- Sustainable palm and palm kernel oil

NOTES

Chapter Two: Sugar

Page

14   Graph calculated by USDA/Center for Nutrition Policy and Promotion. Data last updated Feb. 1, 2014.

17   Graph: Stephen Guyenet and Jeremy Landen, Whole Health Source, Nutrition and Health Science, http://wholehealthsource.blogspot.com.au/2012/02/by-2606-us-diet-will-be-100-percent.html

18   As late as 1963, the average Indian...: 'India's sugar policy and the world sugar economy', FAO (Food and Agriculture Organization of the United Nations) International Sugar Conference, Fiji, August 2012, www.fao.org/fileadmin/templates/est/meetings/sugar_fiji_2012/ADHIRJHA-_India.pdf

18   In 1978 the average rural Chinese...: Zhangyue Zhou et al., *Food Consumption Trends in China April 2012*, report submitted to the Australian Government Department of Agriculture, Fisheries and Forestry, Canberra, 2012, www.daff.gov.au/__data/assets/pdf_file/0006/2259123/food-consumption-trends-in-china-v2.pdf

18   Now their consumption is ten times...: 'China's taste for sugar to send demand soaring', 18 January 2012, www.agrimoney.com/news/chinas-taste-for-sugar-to-send-demand-soaring--4061.html

23   Populations exposed to sugar...: 'Epidemiology of dental disease', Oral Sciences class notes, University of Chicago at Illinois, www.uic.edu/classes/osci/osci590/11_1Epidemiology.htm

24   Binge drinking alcohol...: Vishnudutt Purohit et al., 'Alcohol, intestinal bacterial growth, intestinal permeability to endotoxin, and medical consequences', *Alcohol*, vol. 42, no. 5, August 2008, www.ncbi.nlm.nih.gov/pmc/articles/PMC2614138

24   But if you're like most people...: Richard J Johnson et al., 'Fructokinase, fructans, intestinal permeability, and metabolic syndrome: an equine connection?', *Journal of*

Equine Veterinary Science, vol. 33, no. 2, February 2013, www.ncbi.nlm.nih.gov/pmc/articles/PMC3576823

24   It's early days yet but the science is also increasingly...: S Nasseri-Moghaddam, P Mostajabi and R Malekzadeh, 'Overlapping gastroesophageal reflux disease and irritable bowel syndrome: Increased dysfunctional symptoms', *World Journal of Gastroenterology*, vol. 16, no. 10, 14 March 2010, http://www.ncbi.nlm.nih.gov/pubmed/20222167

25   That fat is stored in the liver...: Maria Maersk et al., 'Sucrose-sweetened beverages increase fat storage in the liver, muscle, and visceral fat depot: a 6-mo randomized intervention study', *American Journal of Clinical Nutrition*, vol. 95, no. 2, February 2012, ajcn.nutrition.org/content/95/2/283.long

26   But left untreated, fatty liver can progress...: KA Lê et al., 'Fructose overconsumption causes dyslipidemia and ectopic lipid deposition in healthy subjects with and without a family history of type 2 diabetes', *American Journal of Clinical Nutrition*, vol. 89, no. 6, June 2009, www.ncbi.nlm.nih.gov/pubmed/19403641

26   There is now interesting scientific speculation...: Sabine Thuy et al., 'Nonalcoholic fatty liver disease in humans is associated with increased plasma endotoxin and plasminogen activator inhibitor 1 concentrations and with fructose intake', *Journal of Nutrition*, vol. 138, no. 8, August 2008, jn.nutrition.org/content/138/8/1452.full

26   But when fructose-derived fat accumulates...: Kimber L Stanhope et al., 'Consuming fructose-sweetened, not glucose-sweetened, beverages increases visceral adiposity and lipids and decreases insulin sensitivity in overweight/obese humans', *Journal of Clinical Investigation*, vol. 119, no. 5, May 2009, www.jci.org/articles/view/37385

27   For most of us, if we ask our body...: Vasanti S Malik et al., 'Sugar-sweetened beverages and risk of metabolic syndrome and type 2 diabetes: a meta-analysis', *Diabetes Care*, vol. 33, no. 11, November 2010, care.diabetesjournals.org/content/33/11/2477.full

27   Along the way, the persistently high blood glucose...: Donald S Fong et al., 'Retinopathy in diabetes', *Diabetes Care*, vol. 27, no. suppl. 1, 2004, care.diabetesjournals.org/content/27/suppl_1/s84.long; *Diabetes: Australian Facts 2008*, Australian Institute of Health and Welfare, Canberra, 2008, www.aihw.gov.au/publications/cvd/daf08/daf08.pdf

28   Graph: NCHS Health E-Stat, 'Prevalence of overweight, obesity and extreme obesity among adults: United States, trends 1960-62 through 2005-2006', Centre for Disease Control and Prevention. NCHS Health E-Stat Prevalence of overweight, obesity and extreme obesity among adults: United States, trends 1960-62 through 2005-2006; LA Helmchen and RM Henderson, 'Changes in the distribution of body mass index of white US men, 1890-2000', Annual of Human Biology, vol. 31, no. 2, March 2004.

28   The average daily food intake has increased...: Agriculture Fact Book, United States Department of Agriculture, www.usda.gov/factbook/chapter2.pdf

29   In other words the blood glucose...: Stanhope, 'Consuming fructose-sweetened, not glucose-sweetened, beverages increases visceral adiposity and lipids and decreases insulin sensitivity in overweight/obese humans'.

29   Just for good measure, fructose also interferes...: Alexandra Shapiro et al.,
      'Fructose-induced leptin resistance exacerbates weight gain in response to subse-
      quent high fat feeding', *American Journal of Physiology: Regulatory, Integrative
      and Comparative Physiology*, 13 August 2008, doi: 10.1152/ajpregu.00195.2008,
      ajpregu.physiology.org/content/early/2008/08/13/ajpregu.00195.2008

29   When fructose is converted to fat...: Sheldon Reiser et al., 'Blood
      lipids, lipoproteins, apoproteins, and uric acid in men fed diets
      containing fructose or high-amylose cornstarch', *American Journal
      of Clinical Nutrition*, vol. 49, no. 5, May 1989, www.ajcn.org/cgi/
      reprint/49/5/832?ijkey=f21115359cab75a94a6228e965f5a7d92134997b

30   And this is likely to be why excess uric acid...: Richard J Johnson et al, 'Is there
      a pathogenetic role for uric acid in hypertension and cardiovascular and renal
      disease?', *Hypertension*, vol. 41, no. 6, June 2003, hyper.ahajournals.org/cgi/
      content/abstract/41/6/1183; Rudolf P Obermayr et al., 'Elevated uric acid increases
      the risk for kidney disease', *Journal of the American Society of Nephrology*, vol.
      19, no. 12, December 2008, jasn.asnjournals.org/cgi/content/abstract/19/12/2407?i-
      jkey=a4a1a77f99ebc2217ec5c4f0009d6086266c8430&keytype2=tf_ipsecsha

30   The number of us requiring treatment...: *Chronic Kidney Disease Hospitalisations
      in Australia, 2000–01 to 2007–08*, Australian Institute of Health and Welfare,
      Canberra, 2010, www.aihw.gov.au/publications/phe/127/11234.pdfx.

30   It's now killing more Australians than either breast or prostate cancer:
      Australian Bureau of Statistics, 'Causes of Death, Australia 2007:
      Diseases of the kidney, urinary system and genitals, (N00-N99)',
      18 March 2009, http://www.abs.gov.au/ausstats/abs@.nsf/0/
      B5C6723470F9A006CA25757C001EF1C1?opendocument

30   And is responsible for one in every seven hospitalisations: Frances Green, Simone
      Littlewood and Claire Ryan, 'Chronic kidney disease hospitalisations in Australia
      2000–01 to 2007–08', Australian Institute of Health and Welfare Canberra
      Cat. no. PHE 127, 2010, http://www.aihw.gov.au/WorkArea/DownloadAsset.
      aspx?id=6442460007

31   A recent British study found that the number of people...: C Kuo, MJ Grainge,
      C Mallen, et al., 'Rising burden of gout in the UK but continuing suboptimal
      management: a nationwide population study', *Annals of the Rheumatic Diseases*.
      15 January 2014.

31   Trial after trial conducted between 1972 and 2005...: Richard J Johnson et al.,
      'Potential role of sugar (fructose) in the epidemic of hypertension, obesity and the
      metabolic syndrome, diabetes, kidney disease, and cardiovascular disease', *The
      American Journal of Clinical Nutrition*, vol. 86, no. 4, October 2007, http://ajcn.
      nutrition.org/content/86/4/899.full

31   Uric acid deactivates nitric oxide...: Christine Gersch et al., 'Inactivation of nitric
      oxide by uric acid', *Nucleosides Nucleotides Nucleic Acids*, vol. 27, no. 8, August
      2008, www.ncbi.nlm.nih.gov/pmc/articles/PMC2701227

31   Recent human studies have conclusively demonstrated...: Clive M Brown et al.,
      'Fructose ingestion acutely elevates blood pressure in healthy young humans',

American Journal of Physiology: Regulatory, Integrative and Comparative Physiology, vol. 294, no. 3, March 2008, ajpregu.physiology.org/content/294/3/R730

32   But when that hypothesis has been put to the test...: James J DiNicolantonio and Sean C Lucan, 'The wrong white crystals: not salt but sugar as aetiological in hypertension and cardiometabolic disease,' Open Heart, vol. 1, issue 1, 2014.

32   But one of the more recent studies...: A Nicolosi et al., 'Epidemiology of erectile dysfunction in four countries: cross-national study of the prevalence and correlates of erectile dysfunction', Urology, vol. 61, no. 1, January 2003, www.ncbi.nlm.nih.gov/pubmed/12559296; E Selvin et al., 'Prevalence and risk factors for erectile dysfunction in the US', American Journal of Medicine, vol. 120, no. 2, February 2007, www.ncbi.nlm.nih.gov/pubmed/17275456

33   As many as one in six Australian women...: WA March et al., 'The prevalence of polycystic ovary syndrome in a community sample assessed under contrasting diagnostic criteria', Human Reproduction, vol. 25, no. 2, February 2010, www.ncbi.nlm.nih.gov/pubmed/19910321

33   A recent Swedish evaluation...: Nathalie Roos et al., 'Risk of adverse pregnancy outcomes in women with polycystic ovary syndrome: population based cohort study', British Medical Journal, vol. 343, 2011, www.bmj.com/content/343/bmj.d6309.abstract

34   The number of IVF treatments...: Bethany Basis, 'IVF Treatments Increased by 50% in Australia and NZ', International Business Times, 10 November 2011, au.ibtimes.com/articles/246670/20111110/ivf-treatments-increased-50-australia-nz.htm

34   In Australia today, approximately one in every 30 children...: 'More IVF babies but fewer multiple births', ABC News Online, 24 September 2009, www.abc.net.au/news/2009–09–24/more-ivf-babies-but-fewer-multiple-births/1440172

34   Low levels of SHBG in women...: Judith S Brand et al., 'Testosterone, sex hormone-binding globulin and the metabolic syndrome: a systematic review and meta-analysis of observational studies', International Journal of Epidemiology, vol. 40, no. 1, February 2011, ije.oxfordjournals.org/content/40/1/189.short

34   It's also well established that people who are obese...: Eric L Ding et al., 'Sex hormone–binding globulin and risk of type 2 diabetes in women and men', New England Journal of Medicine, vol. 361, 2009, www.nejm.org/doi/full/10.1056/NEJMoa0804381

34   But a recent study has shown...: Maria Azrad et al., 'Intra-abdominal adipose tissue is independently associated with sex-hormone binding globulin in premenopausal women', Obesity, vol. 20, no. 5, May 2012, www.nature.com/oby/journal/vaop/ncurrent/full/oby2011375a.html

36   People who have lots of smaller and less fluffy LDL particles...: Benoît Lamarche et al., 'Small, dense low-density lipoprotein particles as a predictor of the risk of ischemic heart disease in men: prospective results from the Québec Cardiovascular Study', Circulation, vol. 95, no. 1, January 1997, circ.ahajournals.org/content/95/1/69.long

36 The most efficient way to convert someone...: Isabelle Aeberli et al., 'Fructose intake is a predictor of LDL particle size in overweight schoolchildren', *American Journal of Clinical Nutrition*, vol. 86, no. 4, October 2007, ajcn.nutrition.org/content/86/4/1174.full; Paul T Williams and Ronald M Krauss, 'Low-fat diets, lipoprotein subclasses, and heart disease risk', *American Journal of Clinical Nutrition*, vol. 70, no. 6, December 1999, ajcn.nutrition.org/content/70/6/949. long

37 Many researchers are now referring to Alzheimer's...: Suzanne M de la Monte and Jack R Wands, 'Alzheimer's Disease Is Type 3 Diabetes–Evidence Reviewed', *Journal of Diabetes Science and Technology*, 2008.

37 A series of recent studies have confirmed that we are two to four times...: Natalie Rasgon and Lissy Jarvik, 'Insulin resistance, affective disorders, and Alzheimer's disease: review and hypothesis', *Journals of Gerontology Series A: Biological Sciences and Medical Sciences*, vol. 59, no. 2, February 2004, biomedgerontology. oxfordjournals.org/content/59/2/M178.abstract

37 One of the recent studies..: Tali Cukierman-Yaffe et al., 'Relationship between baseline glycemic control and cognitive function in individuals with type 2 diabetes and other cardiovascular risk factors: the action to control cardiovascular risk in diabetes-memory in diabetes (ACCORD-MIND) trial', *Diabetes Care*, vol. 32, no. 2, February 2009, http://care.diabetesjournals.org/content/32/2/221. full

37 And the research clearly suggests...: C Carvalho, PS Katz, S Dutta, PV Katakam, Moreira, DW Busija, 'Increased susceptibility to amyloid-β toxicity in rat brain microvascular endothelial cells under hyperglycemic conditions', *The Journal of Alzheimer's Disease*, vol. 38, no. 1, 2014, http://www.ncbi.nlm.nih.gov/pubmed/23948922; Weili Xu et al., 'Mid- and late-life diabetes in relation to the risk of dementia: a population-based twin study', *Diabetes*, vol. 58, no. 1, January 2009, diabetes.diabetesjournals.org/content/58/1/71.full; Paul K Crane et al., 'Glucose levels and risk of dementia', *New England Journal of Medicine*, vol. 369, 2013, www.nejm.org/doi/full/10.1056/NEJMoa1215740

38 Researchers have known for a long time...: Patrick Schloss and D Clive Williams, 'The serotonin transporter: a primary target for antidepressant drugs', *Journal of Psychopharmacology*, vol. 12, no. 2, March 1998, jop.sagepub.com/content/12/2/115.abstract

39 Depression is a major chronic health problem...: *Mental Health Services in Australia 2007–08*, Australian Institute of Health and Welfare, Canberra, 2010, www.aihw.gov.au/publication-detail/?id=6442468381&libID=6442468379&tab=2

39 Fructose is the only carbohydrate...: John Yudkin, 'Dietary factors in arteriosclerosis: sucrose', *Lipids*, vol. 13, no. 5, May 1978, www.springerlink.com/content/5p1348696516v6rl

39 But it does so at the expense of our ability...: JW Crayton, 'Effect of corticosterone on serotonin and catecholamine receptors and uptake sites in rat frontal cortex', *Brain Research*, vol. 728, no. 2, July 1996, www.ncbi.nlm.nih.gov/pubmed/8864491

39   This leads inevitably to fructose addiction...: NM Avena et al., 'Evidence for sugar addiction: behavioral and neurochemical effects of intermittent, excessive sugar intake', *Neuroscience and Biobehavioural Review*, vol. 32, no. 1, 2008, www.ncbi.nlm.nih.gov/pubmed/17617461

40   But new research suggests..: Haibo Liu et al., 'Fructose induces transketolase flux to promote pancreatic cancer growth', *Cancer Research*, vol. 70, no. 15, August 2010, cancerres.aacrjournals.org/content/70/15/6368.abstract

40   It's well established that consistently high blood-glucose levels...: William Faloon et al., 'Elevated glucose increases incidence of breast cancer and brain shrinkage', *Life Extension Magazine*, February 2013, www.lef.org/magazine/mag2013/feb2013_elevated-glucose-increases-incidence-of-breast-cancer-and-brain-shrinkage_01.htm

40   A recent study from the University of California...: Haibo Liu et al., 'Fructose induces transketolase flux to promote pancreatic cancer growth'.

41   But these tests on pancreatic tumours...: Susanna C Larsson et al., 'Consumption of sugar and sugar-sweetened foods and the risk of pancreatic cancer in a prospective study', *American Journal of Clinical Nutrition*, vol. 84, no. 5, November 2006, ajcn.nutrition.org/content/84/5/1171.full; Noel T Mueller et al., 'Soft drink and juice consumption and risk of pancreatic cancer: the Singapore Chinese Health Study, *Cancer Epidemiology, Biomarkers and Prevention*, vol. 19, no. 2, February 2010, cebp.aacrjournals.org/content/19/2/447.abstract

Chapter Three: Polyunsaturated fat
Page

43   Graph: NCHS Health E-Stat, 'Prevalence of overweight, obesity and extreme obesity among adults: United States, trends 1960-62 through 2005-2006', Centres for Disease Control and Prevention, 23 December 2009.

47   Accounted for 86 per cent of the fat consumed in the United States..: YWK Trotter, HO Doty, Jr., WD Givan, and JV Lawler, 'Potential for oilseed sunflowers in the United States', US Department of Agriculture, 1973, http://naldc.nal.usda.gov/naldc/download.xhtml?id=CAT73382700&content=PDF

47   More than 90 per cent of the fat consumed by Americans had come from animals...: David L Call and Ann MacPherson Sanchez, 'Trends in Fat Disappearance in the United States, 1909–65', *The Journal of Nutrition*, 1967, ttp://jn.nutrition.org/content/93/2_Suppl/1.full.pdf

47   In 1925, just 40 in every 100,000 55–64 year old men...: Martha L Slattery and D Elizabeth Randall, 'Trends in coronary heart disease mortality and food consumption in the United States between 1909 and 1980', *The American Journal of Nutrition*, 1998, http://ajcn.nutrition.org/content/47/6/1060.full.pdf

47   By 1950 that number was 600 in 100,000...: ibid.

50   According to US Department of Agriculture statistics...: Economic Research Service (ERS), US Department of Agriculture (USDA), http://www.ers.usda.gov

54   The rate of new prostate cancers in Australia increased...: Australian Institute of Health and Wellbeing, 'Diseases and Injury', *Australia's Health 2010*, http://www.aihw.gov.au/WorkArea/DownloadAsset.aspx?id=6442452954

54   Breast cancer increased by 37 per cent...: ibid.

55   Graph: USDA/Center for Nutrition Policy and Promotion, Feb. 1, 2009.

55   And melanoma increased by 60 per cent in men and 22 per cent in women...: ibid.

57   This has recently been confirmed in research...: Cristian Tomasetti and Bert Vogelstein, 'Variation in cancer risk among tissues can be explained by the number of stem cell divisions', *Science*, January 2015.

58   And we know for certain that in rats...: Adrianne E Rogers, 'Diet and breast cancer: studies in laboratory animals', *Journal of Nutrition*, vol. 127, no. 5, May 1997, jn.nutrition.org/content/127/5/933S.full

58   That's true in the United States...: Jun Wang et al., '5-Lipoxygenase and 5-lipoxygenase-activating protein gene polymorphisms, dietary linoleic acid, and risk for breast cancer', *Cancer Epidemiology, Biomarkers and Prevention*, vol. 17, no. 10, October 2008, cebp.aacrjournals.org/content/17/10/2748.long; Emily Sonestedt et al., 'Do both heterocyclic amines and omega-6 polyunsaturated fatty acids contribute to the incidence of breast cancer in postmenopausal women of the Malmö diet and cancer cohort?', *International Journal of Cancer*, vol. 123, no. 7, October 2008, onlinelibrary.wiley.com/doi/10.1002/ijc.23394/full; Chajès V, 'ω-3 and ω-6 polyunsaturated fatty acid intakes and the risk of breast cancer in Mexican women: impact of obesity status', *Cancer Epidemiology, Biomarkers and Prevention*, vol. 21, no. 2, February 2012, cebp.aacrjournals.org/content/21/2/319. full; Niva Shapira, 'Women's higher risk with n-6 pufa vs. men's relative advantage: an "N-6 Gender Nutrition Paradox" hypothesis', *Israeli Medical Association Journal*, vol. 14, no. 7, July 2012, www.ima.org.il/FilesUpload/IMAJ/0/39/19576. pdf; HJ Murff et al., 'Dietary polyunsaturated fatty acids and breast cancer risk in Chinese women: a prospective cohort study', *International Journal of Cancer*, vol. 128, no. 6, March 2011, onlinelibrary.wiley.com/doi/10.1002/ijc.25703/full; M Gago-Dominguez et al., 'Opposing effects of dietary n-3 and n-6 fatty acids on mammary carcinogenesis: the Singapore Chinese Health Study', *British Journal of Cancer*, vol. 89, no. 9, November 2003, www.ncbi.nlm.nih.gov/pmc/articles/ PMC2394424

58   A randomised controlled trial in US men...: Morton Lee Pearce and Seymour Dayton, 'Incidence of cancer in men on a diet high in polyunsaturated fat', *Lancet*, vol. 297, no. 7697, March 1971, www.thelancet.com/journals/lancet/article/ PIIS0140673671910865/abstract

58   And a similar study in France...: M de Lorgeril et al., 'Mediterranean dietary pattern in a randomized trial: prolonged survival and possible reduced cancer rate', *Archives of Internal Medicine*, vol. 158, no. 11, June 1998, www.ncbi.nlm.nih.gov/ pubmed/9625397

59   One in three Australians...: Tessa K Morgan et al., 'A national census of medicines use: a 24-hour snapshot of Australians aged 50 years and older', *The Medical Journal of Australia*, vol. 196, no. 1, January 2012, https://www.mja.com.au/ journal/2012/196/1/national-census-medicines-use-24-hour-snapshot-australians- aged-50-years-and-older

59   Recent research suggests...: SK Kachhap, P Dange and S Nath Ghosh, 'Effect of omega-6 polyunsaturated fatty acid (linoleic acid) on BRCA1 gene expression in MCF-7 cell line', *US National Library of Medicine*, 2000.

60   The research now clearly shows that the oxidation...: Anne P Toft-Petersen et al., 'Small dense LDL particles - a predictor of coronary artery disease evaluated by invasive and CT-based techniques: a case-control', *Lipids in Health and Disease*, vol. 10, no. 21, 2011, studyhttp://www.ncbi.nlm.nih.gov/pmc/articles/PMC3038964/

62   One in seven Australians over the age of 50 (a little over a million people) has the disease...: Paul Mitchell, 'Eyes on the future: A clear outlook on Age-related Macular Degeneration', Macular Degeneration Foundation, 2011, http://www.mdfoundation.com.au/LatestNews/MDFoundationDeloitteAccessEconomicsReport2011.pdf

62   This number is likely to increase by at least 70 per cent by 2030...: ibid.

63   James Parkinson, surgeon, geologist and palaeontologist...: James Parkinson, *An Essay on the Shaking Palsy*, 1817, Wikipedia, en.wikipedia.org/wiki/File:Parkinson,_An_Essay_on_the_Shaking_Palsy_(first_page).png

64   There, researchers have concluded, annual new cases...: Benjamin CL Lai and Joseph KC Tsui, 'Epidemiology of Parkinson's disease', *British Columbia Medical Journal*, vol. 43, no. 3, April 2001, www.bcmj.org/article/epidemiology-parkinson's-disease

64   Other studies tell us that Parkinson's...: Lonneke ML de Lau and Monique MB Breteler, 'Epidemiology of Parkinson's disease', *The Lancet*, vol. 5, 2006. http://dtfosburgh.pbworks.com/f/Genetic_5.pdf

65   And the number of us with the disease...: Australian Institute of Health and Welfare, 'A snapshot of rheumatoid arthritis', Bulletin 116, May 2013, http://www.aihw.gov.au/WorkArea/DownloadAsset.aspx?id=60129543377

66   Australia doesn't keep good data on any chronic disease...: ibid.

66   About a quarter of RA sufferers...: Access Economics, *Painful Realities: The Economic Impact of Arthritis in Australia in 2007*, Arthritis Australia, Sydney, 2007, www.arthritisaustralia.com.au/images/stories/documents/reports/2011_updates/painful realities report access economics.pdf

66   Alarmingly, it appears that the incidence is increasing...: Australian Institute of Health and Welfare, 'A snapshot of juvenile arthritis'.

66   Researchers have known for some time...: Robert A Lewis et al., 'Leukotrienes and other products of the 5-lipoxygenase pathway – biochemistry and relation to pathobiology in human diseases', *New England Journal of Medicine*, vol. 323, 1990, www.nejm.org/doi/full/10.1056/NEJM199009063231006

66   Analysis of the inflamed synovial membrane...: Emanuela Ricciotti and Garret A FitzGerald, 'ATVB in Focus: Inflammation Prostaglandins and Inflammation', *Arteriosclerosis, Thrombosis, and Vascular Biology*, American Heart Association, 2011, http://atvb.ahajournals.org/content/31/5/986.full

66   Knowing that omega-3 and omega-6 fats act...: Crystal A Leslie et al., 'Dietary fish oil modulates macrophage fatty acids and decreases arthritis susceptibility in mice',

Journal of Experimental Medicine, vol. 162, no. 4, October 1985, www.ncbi.nlm. nih.gov/pmc/articles/PMC2187871

66   That research has led to large numbers of controlled human trials...: Philip C Calder, 'Session 3: Joint Nutrition Society and Irish Nutrition and Dietetic Institute Symposium on "Nutrition and autoimmune disease" PUFA, inflammatory processes and rheumatoid arthritis', *Proceedings of the Nutrition Society*, vol. 67, no. 4, November 2008, www.protherapix.com/documents/provas/rheumatoid arthritis/ PUFA, inflammatory processes and rheumatoid arthritis.pdf

67   In that trial researchers increased the amount of omega-3...: O Adam et al., 'Anti-inflammatory effects of a low arachidonic acid diet and fish oil in patients with rheumatoid arthritis', *Rheumatology International*, vol. 23, no. 1, January 2003, , www.ncbi.nlm.nih.gov/pubmed/12548439

67   We also know that two things in particular...: Anna Mari Lone and Kjetil Taskén, 'Proinflammatory and immunoregulatory roles of eicosanoids in T cells', *Frontiers in Immunology*, 2013. http://journal.frontiersin.org/Journal/10.3389/fimmu.2013.00130/full; X Ma et al., 'A high-fat diet and regulatory T cells influence susceptibility to endotoxin-induced liver injury', *Herpetology*, 2007. http://www.ncbi.nlm.nih.gov/pubmed/17661402

68   We know that omega-6 fats deactivate...: M Takeda and B Soliven, 'Arachidonic acid inhibits myelin basic protein phosphorylation in cultured oligodendrocytes', *Glia*, vol. 21, no. 3, November 1997, www.ncbi.nlm.nih.gov/pubmed/9383037

68   One of the oddest things statisticians have observed..: JF Kurtzke, 'Epidemiology in multiple sclerosis: a pilgrim's progress', *Brain*, 2013, http://www.ncbi.nlm.nih.gov/pubmed/23983034

68   Scientists have known for more...: K Coupland and P Albertazzi, 'Polyunsaturated fatty acids. Is there a role in postmenopausal osteoporosis prevention?', *Maturius*, 2002, http://www.ncbi.nlm.nih.gov/pubmed/12020975; Lauren A Weiss, Elizabeth Barrett-Connor, and Denise von Mühlen, 'Ratio of n–6 to n–3 fatty acids and bone mineral density in older adults: the Rancho Bernardo Study', *The American Journal of Clinical Nutrition*, vol. 81, no. 4, 2005, http://ajcn.nutrition.org/content/81/4/934.long

68   Now new research has thrown light...: 'Omega-6 acids may lead to weaker fish skeleton', FIS Australia, 1 July 2014, http://fis.com/fis/worldnews/worldnews. asp?l=e&country=0&special=&monthyear=&day=&id=69584&ndb=1&df=0

69   One in twenty Australians has osteoporosis...: Osteoporosis Australia Medical & Scientific Advisory Committee, 'What is it?', Osteoporosis Australia, 2014, http://www.osteoporosis.org.au

69   One in four has low bone density...: ibid.

69   In the last ten years the number of GP...: Tomoko Sugiura and Kuldeep Bhatia, 'A snapshot of osteoporosis in Australia 2011', National Centre for Monitoring Arthritis and Musculoskeletal Conditions, April 2011, Australian Institute of Health and Welfare Canberra, http://www.aihw.gov.au/WorkArea/DownloadAsset. aspx?id=10737418747&libID=10737418746

69   A long series of animal studies...: P Albertazzi and K Coupland, 'Polyunsaturated fatty acids. Is there a role in postmenopausal osteoporosis prevention?', *Maturitas*, vol. 42, no. 1, May 2002, www.ncbi.nlm.nih.gov/pubmed/12020975

69   In 2005 researchers at the University of California...: Lauren A Weiss et al., 'Ratio of n–6 to n–3 fatty acids and bone mineral density in older adults: the Rancho Bernardo Study', *American Journal of Clinical Nutrition*, vol. 81, no. 4, April 2005, ajcn.nutrition.org/content/81/4/934.long

70   This latest proof of the bone-destroying power...: 'Omega-6 acids may lead to weaker fish skeleton', FIS Australia, 1 July 2014, fis.com/fis/worldnews/worldnews. asp?l=e&country=0&special=&monthyear=&day=&id=69584&ndb=1&df=0

70   We don't know exactly how omega-6...: M Coetzee et al., 'Stimulation of pros- taglandin E$_2$ (PGE$_2$) production by arachidonic acid, oestrogen and parathyroid hormone in MG-63 and MC3T3-E1 osteoblast-like cells', *Prostaglandins, Leukotrienes and Essential Fatty Acids*, vol. 73, no. 6, December 2005, www.plefa. com/article/S0952-3278(05)00139-0/abstract

72   Rat studies have repeatedly confirmed...: Marc Richard Bomhof et al., 'Fructose during suckling and into weaning promotes increased body weight in young adult rats prior to affecting glucose or fatty acid metabolism', *FASEB Journal*, vol. 21, 2007, www.fasebj.org/cgi/content/meeting_abstract/21/6/A1197-a; Minh Huynh et al., 'Dietary fructose during the suckling period increases body weight and fatty acid uptake into skeletal muscle in adult rats', *Obesity*, vol. 16, no. 8, August 2008, onlinelibrary.wiley.com/doi/10.1038/oby.2008.268/full

72   But an even more recent study has demonstrated...: Ana Alzamendi et al., 'Increased male offspring's risk of metabolic-neuroendocrine dysfunction and overweight after fructose-rich diet intake by the lactating mother', *Endocrinology*, vol. 151, no. 9, 2009, press.endocrine.org/doi/abs/10.1210/en.2009-1353

73   Rat studies performed in the 1970s...: KK Carroll and GJ Hopkins, 'Dietary polyunsaturated fat versus saturated fat in relation to mammary carcinogenesis', *Lipids*, vol. 9, issue 2, 1979, http://link.springer.com/ article/10.1007%2FBF02533866

73   But a truly disturbing study published in 1997...: Leena Hilakivi-Clarke et al., 'A maternal diet high in n-6 polyunsaturated fats alters mammary gland development, puberty onset, and breast cancer risk among female rat offspring', *Proceedings of the National Academy of Sciences*, vol. 94, no. 17, August 1997, www.pnas.org/ content/94/17/9372.short

74   We know that Australian women...: 'Breast cancer in Australia: An overview, 2009', Australian Institute of Health and Welfare and National Breast and Ovarian Cancer Centre, October 2009, http://www.aihw.gov.au/WorkArea/DownloadAsset. aspx?id=6442454634

75   In total, 80 per cent...: TU Sauerwald et al., 'Polyunsaturated fatty acid supply with human milk. Physiological aspects and in vivo studies of metabolism', *Advances in Experimental Medicine and Biology*, 2000.

75   Very recently, a study in humans...: Andrea Estrada, 'Hold the mayo', *The Current: UC Santa Barabara*, 9 September 2014.

75   Omega-6 fats stop us using DHA...: EM Novak, RA Dyer and SM Innis, 'High dietary omega-6 fatty acids contribute to reduced docosahexaenoic acid in the developing brain and inhibit secondary neurite growth', *Brain Research*, October 2008.

76   This confirmed the findings...: William Lassek and Stephen Gaulin, 'Sex Differences in the Relationship of Dietary Fatty Acids to Cognitive Measures in American Children', *Frontiers in Evolutionary Neuroscience*, November 2011.

76   Indeed, one 2011 study...: ibid.

77   One in four Australians now suffers from an allergic..: 'Allergy and Immune Diseases in Australia', Australasian Society of Clinical Immunology and Allergy Inc., 2013. http://www.allergy.org.au/images/stories/reports/ASCIA_AIDA_Report_2013.pdf

77   Reported rates of hay fever, asthma...: ibid

77   Hospitalisation rates for the most extreme...: Woei Kang Liew, Elizabeth Williamson and Mimi LK Tang, 'Anaphylaxis fatalities and admissions in Australia', *The Journal of Allergy and Clinical Immunology*, 28 July 2008, http://www.jacionline.org/article/S0091-6749(08)01929-5/fulltext

77   And the biggest overall change...:ibid

77   Trial after trial has concluded that children...: T Dunder et al., 'Diet, serum fatty acids, and atopic diseases in childhood', *Allergy*, vol. 56, no. 5, May 2001, onlinelibrary.wiley.com/doi/10.1034/j.1398–9995.2001.056005425.x/full; Stefanie Sausenthaler et al., 'Margarine and butter consumption, eczema and allergic sensitization in children. The LISA birth cohort study', *Pediatric Allergy and Immunology*, vol. 17, no. 2, March 2006, onlinelibrary.wiley.com/doi/10.1111/j.1399–3038.2005.00366.x/abstract; E von Mutius et al., 'Increasing prevalence of hay fever and atopy among children in Leipzig, East Germany', *Lancet*, vol. 351, no. 9106, March 1998, www.thelancet.com/journals/lancet/article/PIIS0140-6736(97)10100-3/fulltext

78   This is true in Finnish children...: ibid.

78   Even when the kids themselves aren't...: Stefanie Sausenthaler et al., 'Maternal diet during pregnancy in relation to eczema and allergic sensitization in the offspring at 2 y of age', *American Journal of Clinical Nutrition*, vol. 85, no. 2, February 2007, ajcn.nutrition.org/content/85/2/530.full

78   They've found a very direct relationship...: Malin Barman et al., 'High levels of both n-3 and n-6 long-chain polyunsaturated fatty acids in cord serum phospho-lipids predict allergy development', *Plos One*, July 2013, www.plosone.org/article/info:doi/10.1371/journal.pone.0067920

Chapter Four: Grains and Superfoods
Page

84   According to the Reserve Bank of Australia's...: Philip Lowe, 'World prices and the Australian farm sector', Australian Farm Institute Agriculture Roundtable Conference 2011, Melbourne, 10 November 2011, www.rba.gov.au/speeches/2011/sp-ag-101111.html

84   Graph: ERS Food Availability (Per Capita) Data System (FADS) data set, United States Department of Agriculture Economic Research Service, 4 December 2014,

http://www.ers.usda.gov/data-products/food-availability-(per-capita)-data-system/.
aspx#26715

88   Recent studies have confirmed...: Jody M Randolph et al., 'Potatoes, Glycemic Index, and Weight Loss in Free-Living Individuals: Practical Implications', *Journal of the American College of Nutrition*, vol. 33, issue 5, 2014, http://www.tandfon-line.com/doi/abs/10.1080/07315724.2013.875441#.VMXdokeUdeA; R Sichieri et al., 'An 18-mo randomized trial of a low-glycemic-index diet and weight change in Brazilian women', *The American Journal of Clinical Nutrition*, vol. 86, no. 3, Sept 2007, http://www.ncbi.nlm.nih.gov/pubmed/17823436

88   And one very recent study has found...: Frank M Saks et al., 'Effects of High vs Low Glycemic Index of Dietary Carbohydrate on Cardiovascular Disease Risk Factors and Insulin Sensitivity The OmniCarb Randomized Clinical Trial', *The Journal of American Medicine*, December 2014, vol. 312, no. 23.

91   Approximately half of all US adults and more than 63 per cent of those over 60 regularly take supplements...: K Radimer et al., 'Dietary supplement use by US adults: data from the National Health and Nutrition Examination Survey, 1999–2000', *American Journal of Epidemiology*, vol. 160, no. 4, 15 Aug 2004, http://www.ncbi.nlm.nih.gov/pubmed/15286019

91   43 per cent of all adults regularly using supplements...: ibid.

91   In the year 2000, Australians spent $1.67 billion on dietary supplements...: Australian Institute of Health and Welfare, 'Specialised Mental Health', http://www.aihw.gov.au/WorkArea/DownloadAsset.aspx?id=6442453280

91   This was four times the amount we spent on prescription drugs and triple the amount we spent just seven years earlier...: ibid.

92   Graph: Antioxidant content of a selection of foods: MH Carlsen et al., 'The total antioxidant content of more than 3100 foods, beverages, spices, herbs and supplements used worldwide', Nutrition Journal, vol. 9, paper 3, January 2010, www.nutritionj.com/content/9/1/3

Chapter Five: Why diets (and surgery) don't work
Page

97   The research suggests an obese person...: AG Tsai and TA Wadden, 'Systematic review: an evaluation of major commercial weight loss programs in the United States', *Annals of Internal Medicine*, vol. 142, no. 1, 4 Jan 2005, http://www.ncbi.nlm.nih.gov/pubmed/15630109

97   Almost half the participants...: ibid

98   It's a relatively recent type of diet...: Michelle N Harvie et al., 'The effects of inter-mittent or continuous energy restriction on weight loss and metabolic disease risk markers: a randomised trial in young overweight women', *International Journal of Obesity*, vol. 35, no. 5, May 2011, www.ncbi.nlm.nih.gov/pmc/articles/PMC3017674

98   Studies of the effectiveness of low-carb diets...: Lydia A Bazzano, 'Effects of low-carbohydrate and low-fat diets: a randomized trial', *Annals of Internal Medicine*, vol. 161, no. 5, September 2014, annals.org/article.aspx?articleid=1900694

98   By the twelve-month mark...: Gary D Foster et al., 'A randomized trial of a
      low-carbohydrate diet for obesity', *New England Journal of Medicine*, vol. 348,
      2003, www.nejm.org/doi/full/10.1056/NEJMoa022207

99   That resulted in just 20 per cent of them dropping out...: Lydia A Bazzano,
      'Effects of low-carbohydrate and low-fat diets: a randomized trial', *Annals
      of Internal Medicine*, vol. 161, no. 5, September 2014, annals.org/article.
      aspx?articleid=1900694

99   Like other recent studies on low-fat and low-carb diets...: Bradley C Johnston
      et al., 'Comparison of weight loss among named diet programs in over-
      weight and obese adults: a meta-analysis', *Journal of the American Medical
      Association*, vol. 312, no. 9, September 2014, jama.jamanetwork.com/article.
      aspx?articleid=1900510

99   Associate Professor Traci Mann and her colleagues...: Stuart Wolpert,
      Dieting Does Not Work, UCLA Researchers Report, UCLA
      Newsroom, Los Angeles, 3 April 2007, newsroom.ucla.edu/releases/
      Dieting-Does-Not-Work-UCLA-Researchers-7832

101   Graph: Medicare Item Reports, Department of Human Services, Australian
      Government, https://www.medicareaustralia.gov.au/statistics/mbs_item.shtml

101   In 1993–94, just 550 lap-band...: Medicare Item Reports, Department of Human
      Services, Australian Government.

101   2012–13 this had grown...: ibid

101   Most people are paying the lion's share...: ibid

101   In 2012–13, Australian doctors performed...: ibid

102   About one in five cases require...: Melinda A Maggard et al., 'Meta-Analysis:
      Surgical Treatment of Obesity', *Annals of Internal Medicine*, vol. 142, no. 7, 5 April
      2005, http://www.annals.org/cgi/content/full/142/7/547

106   Between 1980 and 2000...: Australian Institute of Health and Welfare,
      'Overweight and obesity', Australian Government, 2013, http://www.aihw.gov.au/
      overweight-and-obesity/

106   Between 1990 and 2005...: Australian Institute of Health and Welfare, 'Diabetes:
      Australian facts 2008', Australian Government, http://www.aihw.gov.au/WorkArea/
      DownloadAsset.aspx?id=6442454995

106   Between 1985 and 2000...: Australian Institute of Health and Welfare, 'Australia's
      health 2010', Australian Government, http://www.aihw.gov.au/WorkArea/
      DownloadAsset.aspx?id=6442452954

Chapter Six: What to keep and what to buy
Page

126   Graph: Polyunsaturated fat content of popular meats (and a meat substitute):
      NUTTAB (Nutrient tables for use in Australia) 2010 – Australian Food
      Composition Tables, Food Standards Australia New Zealand, Canberra, 2010.

123   But the science has now..: N Shapira, P Weill and R Loewenbach, 'A high n-3
      fatty acid egg vs. a high n-6 fatty acid diet: the significance of health-oriented

agriculture', CABI, http://www.cabi.org/Uploads/animal-science/worlds-poultry-science-association/WPSA-czech-republic-2007/11_Shapira%20Niva.pdf

124   US studies have shown that…: AM Louheranta et al.,'Linoleic acid intake and susceptibility of very-low-density and low density lipoproteins to oxidation in men', *The American Journal of Clinical Nutrition*, vol. 65, no. 5, May 1996, http://www.ncbi.nlm.nih.gov/pubmed/8615351

124   A 2006 review of studies…: ML Fernandez, 'Dietary cholesterol provided by eggs and plasma lipoproteins in healthy populations', *Current Opinion in Clinical Nutrition and Metabolic Care*, vol. 9, no. 1, Jan 2009, http://www.ncbi.nlm.nih.gov/pubmed/16340654

127   Since 1975, Australians have doubled…: *Australia's Seafood Trade*, Department of Agriculture, Canberra, 2013, www.daff.gov.au/__data/assets/pdf_file/0005/2359643/aus-seafood-trade.pdf

128   But now more than half of all fish consumed in Australia…: Department of Agriculture, *The Aquaculture Industry in Australia*, 22 October 2013, www.daff.gov.au/fisheries/aquaculture/the_aquaculture_industry_in_australia

128   In 2010, we maxed out the available supply…: Ian H Pike and Andrew Jackson, 'Fish oil: production and use now and in the future', *Lipid Technology*, March 2010, vol. 22, no. 3, www.iffo.net/system/files/LipidTechpaper-finalpdf.pdf

128   The Australian fish-farming business now proudly boasts…: 'Bred to last', *The Australian*, 18 December 2010, www.theaustralian.com.au/news/features/bred-to-last/story-e6frg8h6-1225971143612

129   Graph: Polyunsaturated fat content of raw Australian seafood: NUTTAB (Nutrient tables for use in Australia) 2010 – Australian Food Composition Tables, Food Standards Australia New Zealand, Canberra, 2010.

136   Graph: Jennifer Di Noia, Defining Powerhouse Fruits and Vegetables: A Nutrient Density Approach, Preventing Chronic Disease, vol. 11, June 2014, doi: 130390, www.cdc.gov/pcd/issues/2014/13_0390.htm

136   It's a question some quite helpful scientists…: Jennifer Di Noia, 'Defining powerhouse fruits and vegetables: a nutrient density approach'.

Chapter Eight: What to expect when qutting sugar.
Page

189   Sadly, the research…: Nicole M Avena, Pedro Rada, and Bartley G Hoebel, 'Evidence for sugar addiction: Behavioral and neurochemical effects of intermittent, excessive sugar intake', *Neuroscience and Biobehavioural Review*, 2008, vol. 32, no. 1, http://www.ncbi.nlm.nih.gov/pmc/articles/PMC2235907/

ACKNOWLEDGEMENTS

You'll have seen me refer to my wife, Lizzie, frequently throughout this book. Clearly she has played a big part in helping our family to undertake a real food lifestyle. She cooks fresh bread four times a week. She makes pizza from scratch once a week (Sunday dinner treat). She batch cooks everything the kids eat at home or take to school and she follows the science voraciously. But her role is much more than that. Lizzie reads every word I write and runs it through the how-on-earth-do-we-do-this-in-practise filter. She tests every recipe and every iteration dozens of times. She researches shortcuts and seeks practical advice from others with a doggedness few possess. So while it seems trite just to acknowledge her, I do, but in the sense that none of this would be remotely possible without her.

Our kids, Anthony, James, Gwen, Adam, Elisabeth & Fin have been, and continue to be, living a real food lifestyle. They have done it (largely) without complaint and with varying levels of commitment to the concept (they have no choice about the practice). Their preparedness to try, and to learn, has been exemplary and well and truly above the call of duty for teenage kids (who don't live in the Middle Ages).

This is the fifth book I have written that has been published by Ingrid Ohlsson (the others were *Sweet Poison, The Sweet Poison Quit Plan, Big Fat Lies* and *Free Schools*). Ingrid has an uncanny knack of knowing when a message is ready to be read. She usually does it in the face of most of the publishing industry telling her she stuffed it up but, with me at least, she hasn't been wrong yet. This book contains information which is, in my view, vital to the health of every person exposed to a Western diet today. It is a message that needs to be very widely read, so I hope Ingrid's legendary nose for a story is right yet again.

Samantha Sainsbury ran the editing at Pan Macmillan and did an exquisite job of walking the fine line between making me feel like I had a say and getting the job done on time. She doubly deserves credit for having to argue with a lawyer (who thinks he's a writer) about whether there was a trademark on the phrase 'Live long and prosper'.

Nicola Young (who also copy edited *Big Fat Lies*) bashed my poorly spelt and appallingly structured manuscript into shape. But more than that, she fact checks like a demon. Over and over I would find her not only questioning the English, but also my interpretation of the science and even whether a particular product did in fact contain a given ingredient. I love that someone with that kind of an eye for detail was looking over my shoulder. She did so much more than edit the copy.

Lastly, my friend and agent Frank Stranges, as usual did nothing (well, all right, he fiddles about with contracts or something), but I suspect will be miffed if I don't acknowledge him.

INDEX

DNA damage 56–8
dopamine 38–9, 63–4, 189
dried fruit 116, 131, 132, 134, 209, 210, 224
drinks 142, 174
  breakfast drinks 213–14
  school lunches 223
drugs 38–9
drusen 63

eating out 171–2
eczema 77–8
eggs 11, 115, 123–5, 296
  breakfast 211, 221
  extra large 229
  poached 210
erectile dysfunction
  fructose, effect of 23, 32–3
exercise 3
extra virgin olive oil 119

fake food 68, 109, 113, 114, 139, 198
  disposing of 114–16
fasting, intermittent 98
fats 6–7, 15, 27
  cheat sheet 118
  cooking fats 204–6
  rules 140–4
  shopping list 305
  smoke point 204–5
  types 44
fatty liver disease 22, 25–6, 35, 89
female infertility
  fructose, effect of 22, 33–5
fibre 130–1
fish 15, 127–30
  farming 127, 128
fish and chips 168
fish oils 66, 67, 69, 75, 92
fish-based products 166–8
flour 115, 148–9
  shopping list 296
food corporations 103–8
food industry 5, 106
fried food 172–5
fried potatoes 160
fructose 19, 22–41, 85, 87, 88, 117, 189
  deleting from diet 100
  fruit, in 130, 133
  harms caused by 22–3
  vegetables, in 135

fruit 7, 11, 15, 115, 120, 130–4
  buying and storing 199–201
  fructose in 130, 133
  school lunches 222, 224
  shopping list 299
fruit juice 21, 116, 131, 134, 137, 192, 224

garlic bread 238–9
gastro-oesophageal reflux disease (GORD) 25
ghee 145, 305
glucose 19, 87, 88, 295
glucose syrup 117, 291, 295
glycemic index (GI) 87–9
goji berries 8, 90, 92
gout 169
  fructose, effect of 23, 30–1
grains 11, 15, 50, 81–4, 148
grapes 120, 132, 134, 209
Greek yoghurt 115, 157, 224, 276
gut, inflamed 23, 24–5

hash browns 162–3, 212
hay fever 77–8
HDL cholesterol 35
heart disease 2, 7, 41–2, 47, 89, 124
  fructose and 22, 23, 35–6
  polyunsaturated fats and 54, 60–2
heartburn 25
high blood pressure, effect of fructose 22, 31–2
honey 19, 20, 85, 116, 117, 149, 160, 209
hot breakfasts 211–13
hot chips 139, 160–2, 163
  recipe 253–5
hunger 95, 98, 196–7
hydrogenation 47
hypertension, effect of fructose 23, 31–2

ice-cream 116, 225, 228, 289
  recipe 291
insulin 27–9, 85
insulin resistance 27–9, 34–5, 37
insulin sensitivity 26
irritable bowel syndrome (IBS) 24
ischemic stroke 35
IVF 33–4

jams 20, 116, 149
  recipe 281–2

kidney disease 89, 169
  fructose, effect of 23, 29–30, 31, 41–2

lactose 17, 117, 141, 142, 156–8, 295
lactose intolerance 157
lamb 51, 123, 296
lap-band surgery 101–2
LDL cholesterol 35–6, 60, 124
legumes 15, 19, 115, 300
lentils 127, 300
leptin 29
Levitra 33
limb amputations 27
lipoproteins 35–6
liver 131
  disease 169
  effect of fructose on 22, 25–6
low-carb diets 98–9
low-fat foods 12, 59
low-GI diets 88–9
lunch 215
lupus 7, 65

macadamia nut oil 305
macadamia nut spread 151, 301
McDonald's 48, 162, 166, 172, 173, 191, 193
macular degeneration 7
  polyunsaturated fats and 54, 62
maltodextrin 117, 295
maltodextrose 117, 295
maltose 117, 295
margarine 7, 12, 48, 59, 74, 78, 106, 116, 127, 144–6, 215, 221
  olive-oil 145–6
mayonnaise 152–5, 215, 301
  recipe 264–5
meal planner 207–8
meal-replacement shakes 97–8
meat 11, 15, 30, 110, 115
  buying and storing 202–3
  marinated 116
  shopping list 296
meat pie 224, 248–50
melanoma 55, 57, 106
Mexican food 182–3
milk 11, 86, 115, 116, 123, 142, 302
  non-dairy 156–7, 304
monounsaturated fats 44, 49
muesli 209, 210, 298–9
multiple sclerosis 7, 65

mushrooms 127, 211, 222
myocardial infarction 35

nervous system, growth of 74–7
nicotine 39, 188
non-dairy milk 156–7, 304
noodles 178
nuts 11, 15, 50, 115, 137–9
  shopping list 300

obesity 2–4, 23, 29, 33, 34, 41–2, 87, 95, 106
  children, in 72–3, 224
  intergenerational transmission 72
oils
  cheat sheet 118
  cold-pressed 119
  extra virgin 119
  labelling 118
  refined 119
  seed 7
  vegetable 6–7
  virgin 118
olive oil 12, 118–19, 130, 164, 305
  margarine 145–6
omega-3 and omega-6 fats 49–53, 54, 56, 58–71, 73–8, 86, 108, 118, 119, 123, 125
opioid drugs 39
osteoarthritis 65
osteoporosis 54, 68–71
oxidation 56–62, 65, 70, 124, 204

'Paleo' diet and lifestyle 82, 85, 98
Palaeolithic diet 82–3
palm oil 52, 143, 163, 164, 305
pancake mixes 212
pancreas 88
  effect of fructose 22, 26–7
Parkinson's disease 7
  polyunsaturated fats and 54, 63–5
party food 225
pasta 87, 216, 270, 297
peanut butter 149–51, 301
pesto 152, 155
pie pastry 251–2
pigs 119, 120, 125–6
pikelets 281–2
pine nuts 52
pizza 175–7
pizza-base recipe 231